Behavioral Objectives — Evaluation in Nursing

Third Edition

Behavioral Objectives — Evaluation in Nursing
Third Edition

Dorothy E. Reilly
Marilyn H. Oermann

National League for Nursing • New York
Pub. No. 15-2367

RT71
R48
1990

This book was set in Goudy by Publications Development Company. The editor and designer was Allan Graubard. Clarkwood Corporation was the printer and binder. The cover was designed by Lillian Welsh.

Printed in the United States of America

Contents

v

About the Authors

Dorothy E. Reilly, EdD, RN, FAAN, is Professor Emeritus, College of Nursing, Wayne State University, Detroit, Michigan.

Marilyn H. Oermann, PhD, RN, is Associate Professor of Nursing, College of Nursing, Wayne State University, Detroit, Michigan.

Preface

Since the first two editions of this book, the world of nursing and the world in which nursing functions have undergone marked change. This third edition is developed to reflect these changes. The original format and intent to demonstrate the relationship between the stated behavioral objectives for an educational experience and the selected evaluation process have not changed; changes have occurred in the contextual framework within which they are discussed.

There are now two authors for this new edition; two nurse educators who share the same philosophical beliefs about the phenomenon of teaching in nursing, but who have their own unique experiences and resources to bring to this presentation.

At this time in our history, questions are being raised as to the appropriateness of using behavioral objectives in a professional educational program because of their perceived rigidity and deterrence to the dynamic processes involved in a teaching–learning experience. An introduction has been added to present the authors' position relative to this question and the rationale for submitting a third edition of this text to our colleagues in nursing education.

This text is more forceful than previous texts in support of the general, open-ended behavioral objectives of Bloom that reflect the human science perspectives of the educational process, particularly as they relate to how individuals learn. The behaviorist model of objective writing, close-ended and specific, with all learning contingencies inclusive to the statement being made, was still very much a part of the educational literature and practice when the earlier editions of this book were published. Although the author at that time noted that these specific objectives had limited use in nursing education, the text did accommodate both styles of writing objectives. The chapters throughout this edition reinforce the original beliefs about the use of open-ended behavioral objectives for setting direction and promoting a sense of fairness, but also develop to a greater degree their implications and potentials for fostering dynamic transformational learning experiences.

In all chapters the text has been updated to reflect the thought and trends of the 1990s and, where indicated, reports of findings from studies conducted since the previous editions are included. In all chapters there has been a significant updating of the recommended readings.

In addition to the introduction, a new Chapter 10 is added, Preparation of Tests Within Nursing Process Framework. This content has been developed at the request of nursing educators to assist them in the preparation of tests for their own clinical content courses in accord with the NCLEX-RN model. Two issues are addressed in this chapter. Suggestions are provided for mapping tests so that there is equity among questions for the stages of the nursing process within the framework suggested by the course objectives. The second element in the chapter relates to the preparation of multiple choice test items for various levels of the cognitive taxonomy for each stage of the nursing process. This chapter in no way suggests that the multiple choice format is the best way to test the cognitive dimension of the nursing process, but it is the method used for licensing examinations for programs preparing individuals for entry into nursing. Because these examinations are given, the chapter is developed to assist faculty in improving the quality of their testing within this structure.

In the belief that faculty skill in preparing behavioral objectives and selecting appropriate evaluation processes is a necessary function of the teaching role, this text is submitted for use by faculty and potential faculty in nursing and other health fields whether teaching in programs in educational institutions, staff development, and continuing or client education. The authors are deeply appreciative of those nursing colleagues who have used previous editions and contributed suggestions for continuing its publication. We hope that the 1990 edition will continue to serve as a meaningful resource to each one of you as you pursue this critical role in nursing.

We are also grateful to our typist, Julia Ploshehanski, who contributed so significantly to the final manuscript.

DOROTHY E. REILLY, EdD, RN, FAAN
MARILYN H. OERMANN, PhD, RN

Preface to the Second Edition

The decision to write a new edition of a book is not taken lightly by the author, for such an endeavor must be supported by the need for new content addressed to increasing knowledge in the area or including new areas that will enrich the book and facilitate its use by the consumer.

This edition incorporates both aspects: some areas are updated while some content is new to the book. The changes reflect feedback from students and colleagues who use the book as well as the author's own experiences in both using the book and conducting workshops and conferences throughout the United States and Canada.

The basic premise of the book remains as stated in the preface of the first edition: "This book deals with the WHAT and the HOW of evaluation with focus on the relationship between these two variables and emphasizes the need for nurse teachers to develop greater creativity and flexibility in their evaluation of the predetermined behavioral objectives." Reviews and comments from users have supported the content of the book and the format by which the content was developed.

One change, however, seemed necessary—that is the change in title. Because the title of the first edition was so lengthy, the book often was referred to as the "one on behavioral objectives," thus negating the true nature of the book, which was to show the relationship between behavioral objectives and evaluation as well as to acknowledge the content relevant to the evaluative process and its strategies. The title selected for the second edition seeks to address this concern.

Major revision of content occurs in four areas of the book: the theory of nursing in Chapter 2; the affective domain in Chapter 4; the principles for preparing multiple recognition items in Chapter 7; and concepts of clinical practice evaluation in Chapter 10. Chapter 4 also includes a list of behavioral terms appropriate for use in writing objectives for all levels of the three taxonomies.

Two new chapters have been incorporated, and Chapter 5 has been augmented by a more specific discussion of the leveling process. Suggestions for program objectives are offered and the process of leveling is presented either by use of the taxonomies or by increasing the complexity of variables with which behaviors are related.

The new Chapter 6 is the result of a need arising from the increased use of continuing education as an update process for practicing nurses. Since the objectives stated for a program are in essence a contract with the consumer, more care needs to be taken to assure that the objectives are relevant and capable of being evaluated.

Chapter 9, which also was added to this edition, resulted from numerous requests by users of the first book. The chapter focuses on the process of test construction, primarily criterion-referenced testing, and illustrates the process for identifying the critical elements or test units within any behavioral objective.

The author is most indebted to students and colleagues who have used the first edition of the book and so generously offered comments and suggestions. It is the hope that this new edition will be even more helpful to individuals participating in the development of and the teaching in educational programs within nursing or other health fields.

DOROTHY E. REILLY

Preface to the First Edition

This book is designed for nursing teachers and for prospective nursing teachers. It aims to help them increase the nursing teacher's competency in the difficult task of evaluating learning achievement, and it maintains that this evaluation process can best be accomplished through the use of behavioral objectives. It is the author's hope that it will prove useful for schools of nursing, for staff development programs whether in hospitals or other health agencies, for continuing education, and for community health education.

The evaluation component of education often can evoke feelings of insecurity, inadequacy, and guilt on the part of nurse educators, especially as they address themselves to the clinical practice portion of the program. Many of these feelings may result from the greater emphasis placed on the HOW of evaluation (procedures to be used) rather than on the WHAT of evaluation (object). Accentuation of methodology over substance has often led to some incongruency between the two, so that evaluation results are invalid in terms of the original intent. Furthermore, failure to identify clearly the object of evaluation has often led to the practice of limiting tests to the evaluation of the cognitive skill of remembering information. Also questionable is the tendency to limit clinical evaluation to skills in technical procedures and to compliance to the behavioral norms of the practice setting.

The current trend toward the use of behavioral objectives as a basis for program development and evaluation has much potential for facilitating the teaching–learning process through the identification of the WHAT.

This book deals with the WHAT and the HOW of evaluation with focus on the relationship between these two variables and emphasizes the need for nurse teachers to develop greater creativity and flexibility in their evaluation of the predetermined behavioral objectives.

The WHAT of evaluation is presented as a discussion of behavioral objectives in nursing in relation to the

1. Derivation to provide for relevancy of these objectives.
2. Development of behavioral objectives. Many books are available for explaining the technique of objective writing; this aspect will receive limited attention.
3. Use of behavioral objectives in a nursing program.
4. Application of the taxonomy of learning behaviors to nursing behaviors.

The HOW of evaluation is presented as a discussion in relation to the

1. Concept of evaluation as derived from one's perspective on the process.
2. Identification of evaluative approaches appropriate to nursing programs.

The two variables—WHAT and HOW—are brought together through the demonstration of

1. Application of each evaluative approach to a specific behavior or to several behaviors.
2. Multi-evaluative approaches for any given specific behavior.

This book is offered in response to requests from my students and from nursing colleagues throughout the country with whom I have shared my ideas and thinking in consultations, institutes, workshops, and other professional forums. These students and colleagues have encouraged me in developing my approach, have challenged me to refine my thinking, and have contributed to my own growth. Indeed, they have been true critics.

Acknowledgment is extended to Margaret Shetland, former Dean at the College of Nursing, Wayne State University, for supporting my endeavors and to those colleagues in the College of Nursing who provided that special type of caring which made the writing of this book a pleasurable and worthwhile experience.

In an endeavor such as writing, the author is enriched by being assisted by individuals who give not only of their expertise, but also of themselves. As this book reaches its final stage of development, I am especially indebted to four such individuals. A special recognition is extended to my dear friend, Hope Brophy, who cast her journalistic eye over the manuscript to insure that it met high editorial standards.

Three individuals, Maria Phaneuf, professor emeritus of public health nursing at the College of Nursing, Wayne State University, LaVaughn Sharp, director of the Grace Hospital School of Nursing in Detroit, and Margretta Styles, Dean of the College of Nursing, Wayne State University, gave unstintingly of their time, humanness, and expertise as readers of the original manuscript. Their thoughtful assessment and constructive criticisms contributed to the refinement of the manuscript.

My deepest appreciation is extended to my mother and to everyone who in his/her own way showed faith in my efforts and provided me with the support necessary for realizing my own dream, the publication of this book.

DOROTHY E. REILLY

Introduction

The call for a curriculum revolution in the 1990s by some nursing educators seeks alterations in philosophy, content, and pedagogy. To many faculty this call seems all too frequent, for developing the "new" curriculum is endemic in many schools and is more a constant than a novel phenomenon. In many instances, however, this change is more a "tinkering" with the curriculum than a substantive change addressed to the preparation of learners for a professional role in a complex, multidimensional society where ambiguity rather than absolutism prevails.

A change is needed, particularly as the vestiges of the training model are removed from our curricula and replaced by educational processes which provide an environment in which learning is viewed as transformation. In this environment faculty and students engage in experience, dialogue, and search for meanings in those issues and practices inherent in nursing practice. Two critical questions raised are: What educational processes are needed? Within what context are they to be offered?

The key element in today's teaching–learning process is interaction whereby participants are involved in those learning experiences fostering skills of problem solving, reflection and critical thinking with real problems. The demands of a rapidly changing society, local, national, and international, can no longer tolerate solutions proposed for a different era. Dissemination of information or show and tell teaching as dominant pedagogical strategies are inappropriate in a professional program preparing practitioners to preserve the human component in care within external forces advocating increased technology, economy efficiency, and unilateral control of the decision-making process. Schön (1983) urges all professional educational endeavors to foster reflective practitioners who go beyond the skill of problem solving to that of problem setting where concerns are identified and the context of addressing them are stated.

New higher level, more complex skills are needed in all domains—cognitive, psychomotor, and affective—by nursing's future practitioners. The issue underlying various proposals for a curriculum revolution relate more to context in which these skills are learned than to the means by which they are attained. A current emphasis expressed by some advocates for change is for greater freedom and flexibility. The structure of our present curricula, patterns, organization, objectives, selected learning experiences, and evaluation are viewed by some as antithetical to the dynamic process needed for transformation to occur. These structures are deemed to be more consistent with a mechanistic concept of nursing reflective of behaviorism. The notion of a structural impediment to dynamic learning challenges the existence of this book, which seeks to describe the relationship between behavioral objectives and evaluation as a means of addressing qualities of accountability, fairness, and efficiency. A fundamental question is: Can the dynamic of transformation in learning occur within a structured curriculum?

Structure is a reality in any educational endeavor and may be external or internal. Before a faculty begins to develop a curriculum, certain structural variables are already in place and require attention. Institutions housing a nursing program have requirements regarding student admission and graduation, course standards, definitions of school term, course length, credit allocation, and evaluation expectations. Increasingly institutions are specifying certain domains of knowledge with which all students must have experience.

Professional programs have their own structural requirements as stated by national accrediting boards, state approval bodies, and licensing authorities. When field practice is a component of a curriculum, practice agencies pose their own structure such as adhering to the mores and values of the agency, availability of practice settings and resources, and times when experience can be accommodated. Since society grants licensure to practice, it too is involved in determining the domain of accountability for practice of those whom it licenses. An increasingly significant outside structural variable also comes from funding agencies who control the purposes for which they grant funds.

Structure is a constant which may be an impediment or may be a facilitator. Some structural factors occur within the nature of the discipline for which a curriculum is proposed.

The body of nursing knowledge is such a variable. Nursing knowledge is not an isolate, but rather a synthesis of nursing theory and practice within the context of a dynamic health care system, or nonsystem, depending on your point of view. Are there certain knowledges and skills expected of any person who is a nurse, a specialized practitioner in nursing, or a leader in the many areas where nursing is evident? How are these knowledges determined by nursing faculty? Can an individual faculty make the decision as to what to teach? How is the teaching of this knowledge planned? How is it sequenced? How is it addressed in terms of the development of a particular student or group of students? These questions are appropriate if transformation is to occur in the learning environment.

There is a logic and rationale to a curriculum plan. Systems theory is relevant to the evolution of a curriculum from the basic philosophical premises on which it is based through all components to its evaluation. This notion of a systematic approach to curriculum planning was first proposed by Tyler in 1950. He identified three domains of learning as relevant to specifying objectives: understanding, skill, and appreciation. However, these terms were not stated as behaviors enabling them to be evaluated. Bloom (1956) refined the domains of knowledge into the following: cognitive, which incorporates intellectual skills; psychomotor; and affective, which incorporates value development and moral reasoning. The objectives are stated in behavioral terms and, like Tyler, are still open ended here with the teaching–learning activities and evaluation strategies left to the province of faculty and students. In 1962, Mager and his colleagues proposed the behaviorist model of objectives, which were specific and included all conditions of learning and criteria for evaluation.

Much confusion centers around the term *behavioral objectives*. Some perceive objectives as derived from the behaviorism model of learning, a natural science theory, and object to its specificity and incompatibility with other theories of learning related to human science such as cognitive, phenomenological, and social. Many who feel that objectives pertain only to low level knowledge have not thought of them within the context of a taxonomy of learning where the highest levels in all learning domains can be stated behaviorally. The objectives proposed by Bloom are presented in a taxonomy format and specify only the behavior expected as an outcome and the knowledge context within which it occurs. The teacher is challenged to be free in selecting learning experiences and evaluation strategies to make the learning experience both substantive and transformational. Lack in the use of the dynamic teaching potentials provided by open-ended objectives are more often than not a function of limitations in the teacher rather than the objectives that were proposed for the experience.

Throughout its three editions, this book has always supported the open-ended approach to objective writing within a taxonomy concept compatible with human science theories. It is the contention of the authors that the problems ascribed to objectives are less associated with the notion of structure and objectives than with their misuse. The content of the book presents the authors' acknowledgment of the significant role of objectives and their use in directing curriculum and in enabling students and faculty to engage in a goal-directed reflective experience.

Bolles (1983) reminds his readers that there are two elements in the future, *change* and *constancy*. Both are important; change represents "challenge, risk taking, adventure at its height, a kind of magic and enhancement lent to our life while constancy represents familiarity, safety, comfort and security" (p. 7). A view of the future incorporating only change provokes anxiety, fear, uncertainty, and powerlessness while one that emphasizes constancy as seen in states of nostalgia, precipitates boredom, inertia, and emotional, mental, and spiritual stagnation. Sister Donley (1989) states, "We cannot blame the Tyler rationale or any organizing framework for all of nursing's curriculum trouble. It has had a positive impact on the quality of nursing education. The strict insistence on measurable objectives backed by the force of law, custom, and accreditation has produced an organized evaluation-oriented system that provides services of reliable quality" (p. 6). The challenge: organization and objectives are constant; more sophisticated use in implementing their intent in accord with the provision of transformational learning is the change.

REFERENCES

Bloom, B. S. (Ed.). (1956). *Taxonomy of educational objectives: Handbook I. Cognitive domain.* New York: Longman.

Bolles, R. N. (1983). Life/work planning: Change and constancy in the world of work. *The Futurist, XVII*(6), 7–11.

Donley, Sr. R. (1989). Curriculum revolution: Heeding the voices of change. In National League for Nursing, *Curriculum revolution: Reconceptualizing nursing education.* New York: National League for Nursing.

Mager, R. (1962). *Preparing educational objectives.* Palo Alto: Fearon.

Schön, D. A. (1983). *The reflective practitioner: How professionals think in action.* New York: Basic Books.

Tyler, R. W. (1950). *Basic principles of curriculum and instruction.* Chicago: University of Chicago.

1

Instructional Accountability

A CURRICULUM FABLE

One time the animals had a school. The curriculum consisted of running, climbing, flying, and swimming, and all the animals took all the subjects.

The Duck was good in swimming, better, in fact, than his instructor, and he made passing grades in flying, but he was practically hopeless in running. Because he was low in this subject, he was made to stay in after school and drop his swimming class in order to practice running. He kept this up until he was only average in swimming. But average is acceptable, so nobody worried about that except the Duck.

The Eagle was considered a problem pupil and was disciplined severely. He beat all the others to the top of the tree in the climbing class, but he used his own way in getting there.

The Rabbit started out at the top of the class in running, but he had a nervous breakdown and had to drop out of school on account of so much make-up work in swimming.

The Squirrel led the climbing class, but his flying teacher made him start his flying lessons from the ground instead of the top of the tree down, and he developed charleyhorses from overexertion at the take-off and began getting Cs in climbing, Ds in running.

The practical Prairie Dogs apprenticed their offspring to a Badger when the school authorities refused to add digging to the curriculum.

1

At the end of the year, an abnormal Eel that could swim well, run, climb, and fly a little was made valedictorian.

(Author unknown)

The highest honors in this school went to an abnormal eel! Are the learners who come out of our programs abnormal eels, that is, abnormal men and women as nurses? What goals direct our programs, what do we evaluate, and what criteria do we use for this evaluation? Can we meet the criterion of accountability for our educational programs?

ACCOUNTABILITY IN EDUCATIONAL ENDEAVORS

Evaluation is a term well known to educators and students in the American society, although its interpretation and impact vary widely among groups and among individuals. Accountability is a term currently used by educators and employed in a sense consistent with its use by many other groups in modern society.

Are the terms *evaluation* and *accountability* synonymous as some references seem to suggest? Both terms connote a process concerned with determining the quality of a substance, action, or event. *Accountability*, however, implies an additional dimension, that of being answerable for quality.

Nursing, along with other professional groups and institutions serving our society, is increasingly held accountable for the quality of service it provides. This entails assessment of goals, resources, actions, and products in light of society's needs and resources.

As nursing teachers in whatever setting we practice, we too will be held more and more accountable for our actions. We must answer to the student, to society, to our profession, to the institution offering the program, and to ourselves.

Society has accepted and legitimized nursing as an institution important to its health care. Is society receiving the nursing care it needs, or is it getting the nursing care we *think* it needs or deserves? Where is the consumer of our services fitting into deliberations on the kind of nursing for which we are preparing practitioners? As educators, we must respond to society's concern about the rising cost of preparing nurses. Can we demonstrate that the nurses sent into the health care system have made a difference for the better in the quality of health care provided in proportion to the scope of their educational preparation?

The rapidity of change within all subsystems of our society challenges nursing to make its own changes so that its participation in the health delivery system is compatible with society's needs and nursing's areas of expertise. As educators, are we contributing to goal setting, implementation, and evaluation of nursing's contribution toward society's health? Are our educational programs consistent with these goals and will our graduates be prepared to practice accordingly?

The institutions or agencies to which we belong must also meet the test of accountability to their governing bodies and to society. What responsibilities do nurse teachers assume in participating in the formulation of philosophy and goals, in program planning and development, and in evaluating attainment of goals? To what extent are our own areas of control developed in concert with the goals of the institution?

The student, our direct consumer, is the pivotal person in our educational programs. Is the student getting the kind of program that is needed or is the program the one *we think* is needed or deserved? Are we asking the student to be an "abnormal eel" or a healthy vibrant learner? Where does the student fit into deliberations about the program of studies? How well do we meet our contract with the learner?

Do our educational offerings stand the test of accountability? We as nurse teachers have been entrusted by society and by our profession with the responsibility to lead and to shape nursing. We are the gatekeepers of our profession, with the power to determine who enters the profession and to define the nature of nursing practice. How well are we using the power bestowed on us?

How well do we meet the test of accountability to ourselves? Are we authentic individuals? Have we formalized for ourselves values and beliefs that guide our actions? Are we true to those values, and are we real and genuine human beings?

The questions are raised here to remind nursing educators involved with the development and evaluation of nursing programs that they must incorporate the concepts of relevance and responsibility for quality in any plan for accountability.

RELATIONSHIP OF BEHAVIORAL OBJECTIVES TO ACCOUNTABILITY

Throughout much of the history of education, educational objectives have been an integral part of program planning. For the most part, objectives have been generalized statements that did not lend themselves readily to operationalization in the curriculum nor to meaningful evaluation. Two movements have influenced educators to recognize the need for greater specificity and clarity in statements of objectives:

1. The development of programmed instruction.
2. Society's mandate for professional accountability.

The development of programmed instruction and instructional technology demonstrated the need for a more precise statement of objectives, so that the focal point of learning could be defined more sharply and the feedback evaluation made more specific.

Demand for accountability of educational endeavors now makes it necessary that students' learning evaluation be related to instructional goals and efforts. This means that instructional accountability within our society has been shifted somewhat from the student to the instructor. This shift requires that clearly and precisely stated objectives must be used as a basis for determining accountability.

Behavioral objectives, unlike content objectives, are more amenable to evaluation. They are statements that describe the behavior the student is expected to exhibit as a result of one or more learning experiences. Emphasis on behavior means that evaluation is concerned with what the student does rather than on the "material covered," as is typical of content-oriented objectives.

The identification of behavior as the critical variable in the evaluation process arises from the concept of the learning process. Learning is described as a change in behavior as a result of "experiencing." Education is charged with expediting a student's learning by selecting experiences that foster the desired change in behavior. Therefore, selection of behaviors appropriate to a learning situation and their statement in measurable terms give direction to the learner's experiences and become the object of student evaluation.

INFLUENCE OF BEHAVIORAL OBJECTIVES ON THE TEACHING–LEARNING PROCESS

The teaching–learning process is a human interaction that has been taking place since the origin of the human race. Once limited to meeting survival needs within a sharply defined cultural group, it now relates not only to an individual's survival needs, but to the search for meaning in a complex pluralistic society. Pressures exerted on this interaction are constant, varied in intensity, and often dichotomous in nature. Each human being entering this interaction is surrounded by a particular life space or "bubble," which is unique to each and into which ideas, feelings, and values are selectively admitted.

The fragility of this interaction requires that educators provide the climate that assists participants toward mutual fulfillment. It is apparent in this complicated society that interactions among individuals depend on clear communication for effectiveness. This clarity of communication is most important when the teacher and learner meet, especially since a change in behavior is the expected outcome.

Behavioral objectives serve as a vital source of communication to all involved in this human interaction, without regard to whether concern is with a total nursing program or an individual learning experience. When the intent (expected behavior) is "on the table," there is little need for the learner to "psych out" the instructor. Since any given goal is clearly identified, all participants are able to channel their energies in the same direction. Not only does this result in maximal student learning, but it also promotes the climate of trust essential to the teaching–learning process carried on as a shared enterprise. Lowman (1984) addresses the importance of sharing with the students at the beginning of the experience the objectives that have been prepared. Such discussion helps students to see where they are heading in this experience and its importance in the whole educational plan. The students are more likely to meet expectations if these are clearly stated well in advance (p. 152).

Because our society is changing constantly, it is incumbent upon us, as educators, to assist the learner in accepting goal-directed learning as a lifelong process. Since this implies accepting responsibility for one's own learning, our programs must provide sufficient learning experiences to internalize this value. Behavioral objectives offer students the opportunity to become self-directing. When the goals are clear, students can direct their own endeavors toward activities that will assist them in achieving these goals.

Behavioral objectives also discipline educators in their responsibilities as teachers. They force them to be clear and precise in communicating their intent. Objectives direct the selection of priorities in teaching and learning activities and help faculty to identify the trivia that may have been cluttering the educational experience. Behavioral objectives require instructors to be informed about *content* and *process*, as implied in the objectives. Most significantly, perhaps, they require teachers to meet their contracts with students. They state what is expected of the learner and direct faculty to provide the kind of program that will facilitate the attainment of that behavior.

INFLUENCE OF BEHAVIORAL OBJECTIVES ON THE EVALUATION PROCESS

Evaluation has been a part of the teaching–learning process since that process began. At one time, its focal point lay within a utilitarian framework; it answered the question: Is it useful? Today, there is not one focal point but many foci, as teachers deal with the complexity of an individual's response to the environment. Whereas historically educators made mental discipline the object of evaluation, today they are concerned with the learner as a whole being in an almost infinite variety of circumstances.

The evaluation process will be discussed further on in the book, but it is important to the discussion of objectives, at this point, to present one concept of evaluation. Nurse educators have asked repeatedly for a means for objective evaluation. The search has been pursued in many directions. (The impossible quest!) If one looks carefully at the word, one can see why objective evaluation alone is unattainable. The work e(valu)ation contains the word *value*, which connotes a personal choice.

Therefore, anyone looking to behavioral objectives as a means of providing for *objective* evaluation will be disappointed. The very selection of the behaviors to be evaluated, whether selected by one person or many, is a personal choice.

Behavioral objectives, by their clarity, communicate the expected behavior signifying the learner's achievement. Thus, the evaluator and the evaluatee know the behavior to be appraised. The element of the unexpected has been eliminated, and the learner does not need to direct energy toward trying to determine "what the test will be about." Although evaluation cannot be objective, it can be *fair*. Fairness in evaluation is a necessary prerequisite to a learning environment that fosters student growth.

Many nurse educators stress the need for nursing students to evaluate themselves, as evaluation must be an on-going process throughout professional lifetimes. Because behavioral objectives are designed to foster performance in terms of goals, the students possess a means for evaluating their own progress and organizing their efforts into relevant activities.

Behavioral objectives also discipline educators as to their evaluation responsibilities. They not only request a clear statement of what the student is to learn, they also challenge appropriate evaluation of that learning. They compel teachers to evaluate only what they have stated as their intent, thus precluding the inclusion of extraneous material. Of particular importance is adherence to evaluation of stated behavior. How often has a behavior been stated as *analyzing* a phenomenon while the test question asks the student to *list* a certain number of characteristics of the phenomenon? Analyzing and listing are not the same intellectual behaviors.

ARGUMENTS AGAINST BEHAVIORAL OBJECTIVES

Behavioral objectives are not a panacea for all educational ills. Some educators do not even see them as significant to teaching and learning and regard their preparation as a pedagogic exercise. Most faculty have some objectives for their courses, but in some instances these objectives remain in the files, are available only on request, and have little relevance to the actual learning situation.

As a basis for this discussion, it is important to clarify the meaning of educational objectives. Educational objectives are used to identify intended behavioral outcomes of the educational process whether for an individual experience or a total program of studies. The acceptance of the behavioral response is predicated on the concept that learning, as an outcome, is manifest by a change in behavior which is either observable or inferred by a resulting product. The latter relates to the intellectual skills which can not be observed directly, that is, the skill of analysis is evident in a written or oral presentation of a situation which has been analyzed in accord with principles of logic, critical thinking, and possibly intuition.

Educational objectives do not refer to another concept of learning, the process by which knowledge becomes integral to the functioning of an individual. The use of the term *behavioral* as a modifier for objectives denotes that they are action-oriented rather than content-oriented. The specific action is always contextual relative to a body of knowledge.

Teachers of nursing have raised several arguments against behavioral objectives that are important for us to consider. There is no intent to deal with the issues in depth here, but perhaps this book will provide the rationale for further discussion. Five common arguments against behavioral objectives are:

1. Behavioral objectives are derived from behaviorism, a natural science of learning, and thus are incompatible with other learning theories from the human sciences such as cognitive, social, or phenomenological.

2. Predetermined objectives express the teacher's expectation of the outcome and do not provide an opportunity for the student to seek own objectives.

3. They interfere with the freedom to learn and teach and thus stifle the creative process.

4. Their precision is incompatible with a complex field of study such as nursing.

5. They require more time for development than is warranted by their effect in the program.

1. Behavioral Objectives—Behaviorism

The selection of objectives for any educational endeavor reflects the philosophy of education and theory of learning accepted by a faculty. Program objectives are congruent with the beliefs of the faculty as a whole in terms of the stated mission of the institution and the processes by which it is fulfilled.

It is important to discriminate between the terms *behaviorism* and *behavior*, however. Behaviorism, as used in education, relates to the specific theory of learning which stresses the direct relationship between stimulus and response as noted in the paradigm, S——R. Other theorists use a different paradigm, S——O——R based on the belief that the process of learning does not entail a direct linkage between stimulus and response, but rather the individual (organism) interprets and acts upon the stimulus in accord with own experiences, values, and meanings. The term *behavior* is a response phenomenon to one or more stimuli and thus can be used in describing the outcome of learning with any theoretical position.

Objectives written in the behaviorism mode are closed-ended; that is, they include all the conditions of learning and evaluation. These statements are consistent with the belief that all environmental contingencies are controlled and reinforcement in learning is directed at a response predetermined to be "good" or "right." Behavioral objectives for other theories of learning are open-ended by specifying only the behavior to be attained and the knowledge context in which it occurs. The conditions of learning and evaluation are functions of the choice of teacher and/or learner.

MacDonald and Wolfson (1971) note that when the concept of behavioral objectives was proposed they foretold a promising development in curriculum development which at that time was content driven emphasizing rote memory. The notice of action on the part of the learner was most welcome. They perceived the behavior as part of the whole process of a stimulus situation, a unique individual capable of selecting and interpreting the meaning of the situation in light of own experience and observable performance (p. 120). It is the specificity of the objectives that has altered their intent. The use of the term *behavioral objectives* implies behaviorism when all the conditions of learning and evaluation are specified. Mager (1962), Tanner (1972), and others prescribe to this specific approach, and many competency-based programs are derived from this view. The open-ended objectives can be used with any theory of learning that conceptualizes the learner as an active participant in the process. Educators who prescribe to this approach to objective writing are Bloom (1956); Krathwohl, Bloom, and Masia (1964); Reilly and Oermann (1985); and others.

2. Teacher Preparation of Objectives

This concern relates to who should prepare educational objectives and when should they be stated. Kliebard (1975) dislikes the product implication of objectives. "A curricular objective in this sense is only a way of stating what someone will do or behave like once we get through with him" (p. 46). MacDonald and Wolfson (1971) express displeasure with the behaviorism model. Behavioral objectives, they state, specify that the teacher's view in-clude all the contingencies of learning, thus leaving out consideration of individual differences among learners.

Bloom (1956) supports the position that objectives prepared by teachers reflect a conscious choice based on their own experiences and the use of vari-ous kinds of relevant data. Lowman (1984) challenges the notion that students should formulate their own objectives for such activity fails to capitalize on the expertise of the instructor and can waste precious time on the part of the learner. Bevis (1989), in recognition of the practice component of nursing edu-cation which implies activity, supports the notion of faculty stated objectives. "It behooves nursing educators to spell out objectives behaviorally on all levels" (p. 182).

There is a tendency to approach this matter of teacher–student initiated objectives from an either/or position when in reality circumstances enable both practices to occur. The nature of the knowledge or skill to be learned, the readiness and experience of the learner, the time allocation for the experience, and the opportunity for extraneous learning to occur all influence the deci-sion as to who will prepare the objectives. Bloom (1982) conducted research to determine cognitive and affective entry characteristics which connote a learner's readiness to engage in certain learning tasks. The characteristics of intelligence and aptitude are acknowledged as readily stable characteristics while others are alterable and become the objectives of the teaching.

Diekelmann (1989) expresses concern regarding the inequality in power between teacher and learner and advocates the empowerment of the student. No doubt, such inequity is a reality, for the instructor is the expert in the field. This is especially true in a professional field such as nursing where knowledge is highly specialized and where the faculty must possess knowledge and the vision of the field not only bounded by the present, but which is universal and future-directed. Diekelmann's study population is composed of adult learners who are practitioners in the field reentering formal studies to acquire a degree in nursing. That is a group who appropriately should be empowered to have more involvement in the setting of objectives within those designated for the program. It is important that empowerment of students to direct their experi-ence is not at the expense of the rightful empowerment of the teacher.

Well-stated objectives reflect the teacher's expertise, and teaching proto-cols are directed toward enabling students to search for knowledge in terms of own meanings. The program for educating the nurse moves from the initial teacher selection of knowledges within the domain of nursing which are then articulated into objectives to the student's identification of knowledge domains significant for practice of own competency and articulation of appropriate objectives. There has been reference in the literature to the teacher-selected structure as signifying a training education model, rather than a professional model. This is a perception which reflects the concept of objectives as limited to lower level competencies. However, the processes of education are altered in accord with increased behavioral expectations as the learner's abilities evolve and learning is perceived as a dynamic process of transformation compatible with professional education.

The perception that teacher-prepared objectives are directed at lower level competencies is a fact. One need only look at the objectives stated for continuing education programs or conferences to concur with this perception. This is an example of misuse of behavioral objectives, for when they are written within a taxonomy framework, the specific level of competency to be attained can be so stated. The preparation of behavioral objectives expressed at various taxonomy levels is the major focus of this book and will be dealt with in more detail later.

3.   Behavioral Objectives—Freedom to Teach and Learn

Another argument declares that behavioral objectives, which state the anticipated result of the learning experience, restrict the freedom and creativity of the teacher and learner. This hypothesis arises, perhaps, from a misunderstanding of the use of objectives in a program of study. Behavioral objectives provide a framework from which a program, learning experience, or evaluation method can be developed. Structure, if relevant and flexible, does not stifle freedom but rather provides for it. One need only be a part of a blackout, such as New York experienced in 1965, to realize how necessary the structure of a network of traffic lights at street intersections is to the flow of traffic to a designated route or goal. Without the structure (lights), traffic halted at intersections until outside intervention became necessary. So, too, without the structure provided by behavioral objectives, learner and teacher may become immobilized at the intersection waiting for outside intervention. This delay may be costly in terms of time, and one cannot ignore the pressures of time on all individuals and the consequent responsibility of the educational endeavor to expedite the learning process.

Although the goal is defined, there is much opportunity for the teacher and learner to be creative in developing ways of meeting it. A stated goal does not mean that all learners and teachers must "march to the same drummer": it does mean that once a goal has been established, participants are free to find their own drummers.

The behaviorism modality for writing objectives has fostered the notion that no alternatives exist since all conditions of learning are stated. In reality, this observation is true; the objectives are viewed as absolutes and the learning environment becomes stifled. However, open-ended objectives, rather than being restrictive, challenge the teacher and learner to engage in a dynamic experience and avail themselves of the multiple ways of meeting objectives. Teachers impose much of their perceived rigidity on themselves, often because moving from the known makes them vulnerable and requires more risk-taking than they are accustomed too. Concern for acceptance by or approval from others in the situation such as colleagues, students, practitioners in the setting, or educational administrators can become a significant impediment to creative teaching. Blame for lack of creative teaching is then directed toward the objectives for the experience. Acceptance of the challenge offered by open-ended objectives leads the teacher and student into the essence of the experience relative to the student's readiness to find meaning. In such an experience, often more learning results than was anticipated by the objectives; such learning needs to be acknowledged and related to the total learning experience. Drummers find their own meaning when they are free within themselves to search. Lowman (1984) reminds us of the responsibility of the teacher in regard to objectives. "Although thoughtful selection of content and objectives contributes significantly to a course, still, as in warfare and athletics, the value of a battle or game plan depends most on how well it is executed and whether it is flexible when surprises occur" (p. 146).

4.   Behavioral Objectives—Complexity of Nursing

In an argument against the use of behavioral objectives, some faculty members suggest that the requirement for precision in behavioral objectives is inconsistent with the nature of nursing practice, which is by definition quite complex. The belief is that emphasis on particulars leads to compartmentalization of nursing practice, an unmanageable quantity of nursing behaviors, and emphasis on lower level behaviors.

Nursing knowledge is not content bound. It includes multiple cognitive, psychomotor, and affective competencies through which the nurse is able to respond to a practice role in a micro and macrosystem of health care delivery. The role incorporates responsibility in a community-directed as well as a professionally-directed activity. Research by Benner (1984) has portrayed the multidimensional role of our practice within the clinical settings. At the same time, nursing is moving into other role demands as it enters more intensely the social, political, and economic venues. In these areas leadership skills in autonomy, advocacy, and collaboration are required within the context of caring, humanistic professionals.

Is the development of such competencies incompatible with the concept of behavioral objectives? Their multiplicity and complexity suggest that there be an even greater necessity for objectives so that a selective, integrative, and developmental process can occur. All these competencies have a similar basis in nursing knowledge as well as the specific knowledges which underlie their functioning. Such competencies can be written as open-ended behavioral objectives which guide their development in an evolving process. This process includes the higher level behaviors compatible with those in the taxonomies and need to be stated at the appropriate place in the curriculum and in the level of the program.

5. Behavioral Objectives—Time Demand

This argument suggests that the development of behavioral objectives is a time-consuming process, the cost benefit of which does not justify the amount of time it requires. Perhaps one needs to consider the perspective one brings to the task of delineating objectives. Is it viewed as a mechanical task or a synthesizing process? Experience has indicated that as faculty members become involved in the process of developing behavioral objectives, they explore their own knowledge, values, and beliefs about the entire spectrum of teaching and learning; about nursing; about their society; and about themselves. Behavioral objectives represent a synthesis of such explorations so that their follow-through (objectives into the program) is expedited quickly. Therefore, time spent is not in terms of pedagogical demand; rather it represents a thoughtful deliberation relative to the knowledge requirements, the level of skill in using the knowledge, and the evolutionary process in meeting the desired competency.

OVERVIEW

This book supports the contention that carefully stated objectives are essential, providing direction for program planning and evaluation. It is not addressed to the total process of curriculum development and the many-faceted aspects of evaluation.

Goal-setting for any educational experience is as much a responsibility of the learner as of the teacher. Mutual respect for each other's objectives and a concerted effort to blend the two sets of objectives into a common set of goals provide for an educational experience that is both developmental and fulfilling.

In any program evaluation, accountability must be directed toward several components: the evaluation of student performance, the process used, and the rightness and completeness of goals. It must also be recognized that some evaluation may not be directly related to a stated goal; that is, there may be goal-free evaluation as well as goal-directed evaluation.

The teaching–learning dynamic is a human interaction process where participants bring their own frame of reference—experiences, values, motivations, and knowledges—to give meaning to the experience. Thus, often the outcome of such an interaction may result in varied meanings for individuals. Although the experience is directed primarily toward a specific goal attainment, other serendipitous learnings may result. Such unanticipated learnings are most significant in the development of the learner and need to be acknowledged in the evaluation. There is no place for absolutism in using objectives. They are guides which lead toward desired goals, but learning cannot be confined and objectives will not necessarily be all inclusive. Therefore, the teacher must be as alert in any situation to the unanticipated as the anticipated learning outcomes.

Nonetheless, this book focuses primarily on the relationship between behavioral objectives and evaluation. Its aim is to assist the nurse teacher in acquiring congruence between stated goals of instructional endeavor and the quality of strategies used to determine the degree to which the learner has attained those goals.

SUMMARY

Accountability for the quality of an educational endeavor has shifted from the learner to the teachers. In nursing, the teachers are accountable to the students, to society, to the institution providing the program, to the profession, and to themselves.

Behavioral objectives that identify the behavior the learner is expected to exhibit as a result of one or more learning experiences provide a basis for ascertaining accountability.

The specificity of objectives is determined by the underlying theory of learning: closed-ended with all the conditions of the learning experience included as in behaviorism or open-ended with only the behavior within the context of the knowledge domain as appropriate for such human science theories as cognitive, social, and phenomenological. Open-ended objectives within a taxonomy format are most pertinent for a professional program such as nursing. With the processes of the educational experience unstated in the objective, the students and teachers are free to select those learning experiences which foster an interchange and growth among the participants. The result of such an interaction nurtures the growth of the learner into a knowledgeable, competent, reflective practitioner for a rapidly changing profession and society.

Some arguments have been proposed against the use of objectives. In general, they object to the perceived close association of objectives to behaviorism, the assumption of teacher direction at the expense of the student's needs, the felt impediment to creativity, and the inconsistency of specific objectives to nursing's real complexity.

Many of the arguments against the use of objectives arise from their misuse or a misunderstanding of the role of objectives in the total educational process. The following chapters will address many of these areas of confusion and demonstrate that behavioral objectives are relevant to the multifaceted domain of nursing knowledge. When they are prepared within a taxonomy format, they can foster the evolutionary process of the formation of a nurse throughout the various stages of development.

REFERENCES

Benner, P. (1984). *From novice to expert: Excellence and power in clinical nursing practice.* Menlo Park, CA: Addison-Wesley.

Bevis, E. O. (1989). *Curriculum building in nursing: A process* (3rd ed.). New York: National League for Nursing.

Bloom, B. S. (Ed.). (1956). *Taxonomy of educational objectives. Handbook I: Cognitive domain.* New York: Longman.

Bloom, B. S. (1982). *Human characteristics and school learning.* New York: McGraw-Hill.

Diekelmann, N. L. (1989). The nursing curriculum: Lived experiences of students. In National League for Nursing, *Curriculum revolution; Reconceptualizing nursing education* (pp. 25–42). New York: National League for Nursing.

Kliebard, H. M. (1975). Persistent curriculum issues in historical perspective. In W. Pinar (Ed.), *Curriculum theorizing: The reconceptualists* (pp. 39–50). Berkeley: McCutchan.

Krathwohl, D. R., Bloom, B. S., & Masia, B. B. (1964). *Taxonomy of educational objectives. Handbook: Affective domain.* New York: Longman.

Lowman, J. J. (1984). *Mastering the techniques of teaching.* San Francisco: Jossey-Bass.

MacDonald, J. B., & Wolfson, B. J. (1971). A case against behavioral objectives. *Educational Digest, 37*(22), 119–128.

Mager, R. T. (1962). *Preparing educational objectives.* Palo Alto: Fearon.

Reilly, D. E., & Oermann, M. H. (1985). *The clinical field: Its use in nursing education.* Norwalk, CT: Appleton-Century-Crofts.

Tanner, D. (1972). *Using behavioral objectives in the classroom.* New York: MacMillan.

RECOMMENDED READINGS

Bigge, M. L. (1982). *Learning theories for teachers.* New York: Harper & Row.

Eble, K. E. (1973). *Professors as teachers.* San Francisco: Jossey-Bass.

Eble, K. E. (1988). *The craft of teaching* (2nd ed.). San Francisco: Jossey-Bass.

Gagne, R. (1972). Behavioral objectives? Yes. *Educational Leadership, 30,* 394.

Hammack, F. N. (1982). Education for nursing: Problems and prospects. *New York Educational Quarterly, 13*(2), 8–14.

Kibler, R., Barker, L., & Miles, D. (1970). *Behavioral objectives and instruction.* Boston: Allyn & Bacon.

King, I. M. (1986). *Curriculum and instruction in nursing.* Norwalk, CT: Appleton-Century-Crofts.

Kitchner, K. S. (1983). Educational goals and reflective thinking. *Educational Forum, 47*(5), 75–79.

Kliebard, H. M. (1975). Reappraisal: The Tyler rationale. In W. Pinar (Ed.), *Curriculum theorizing: The reconceptualists* (pp. 70–83). Berkeley: McCutchan.

Reilly, D. E. (1981). Why objectives? Relationship to occupational health nursing practice. *Occupational Health Nursing, 29*(1), 7–11.

Schön, D. A. (1983). *The reflective practitioner: How professionals think in action.* San Francisco: Jossey-Bass.

Schön, D. A. (1990). *Educating the reflective practitioner.* San Francisco: Jossey-Bass.

Scriven, M. (1972). Pros and cons about goal-free evaluation. Evaluation comment. *Journal of Educational Evaluation, 3:*1.

Yager, S. J. (1971). Behavioral objectives: Where and where not. *Kappa Delta Pi Record, 8,* 99.

2

Derivation of Behavioral Objectives

Two processes are involved in the development of behavioral objectives: one relates to their derivation and is addressed to the substance, the other relates to the writing and is addressed to the prescription for the technique. To ensure significant input, participants in the development of these objectives should include representation from those directly involved with the program or learning experience, such as nurse-educators, consumers (nursing students, graduate nurses, patients, families, community groups), administrators, and experts in the subject matter.

The first process is a critical one in meeting the criteria of relevancy and responsibility for quality. Educational programs do not occur in a vacuum, but are always part of the teachers' and learners' total life experiences as well as those of the groups and society to which they belong. Failure to deal with this fact when developing behavioral objectives for a program leads to objectives limited in scope, inconsistent or unrealistic in behavioral expectations, and difficult if not impossible to evaluate. The derivation of substance then must include not only knowledge of subject matter of the discipline to be learned, but it must also include a knowledge of society and the professional as it relates to the program as well as the participants' values, attitudes, and beliefs about the nature of person, the learner, and the teaching–learning process in which all are involved.

Three steps are included in this derivation process. In the first step, participants explore their knowledges, values, beliefs, and attitudes relative to the seven areas depicted in Figure 2–1:

17

1. Nature of person
2. Societal goals and trends
3. Professional goals and trends
4. Nature of the learner
5. Concept of the teaching–learning process
6. Philosophy of the agency offering the programs
7. Models of nursing.

There is no order of priority for these areas of investigation, thus they are represented as circular phenomena around the objective. Belief about the nature of person transcends all other areas, and thus is depicted as a circle through

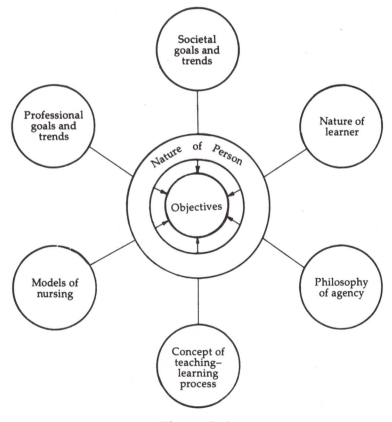

Figure 2–1
Source of Objectives Model

which all other areas transect. The question to be asked in the exploration of these areas and the direction to be pursued in seeking answers will depend upon the nature of the program to be developed.

In the second step, the participants identify from their exploration of these areas the concepts, ideas, theories, and values pertinent to the learning situation. Synthesis is the last step of the process. Here the *What* of behavioral objectives is clarified.

The rest of this chapter identifies some of the matters under each of these areas that have particular bearing on behavioral objectives for a nursing program. The identification is by no means extensive, but hopefully it will provide clues that will give direction to the thinking of groups concerned with the development of behavioral objectives.

NATURE OF PERSON

An exposition of a group's concept of the nature of person is not only important as a basis for the teaching–learning interaction, but it is vital to the development of a conceptual framework for any program related to the helping process. Nursing (as well as medicine, ministry, social work, teaching) is among the groups identified as a helping profession; thus the nature of its practice is the service to human beings. Behaviors that characterize that practice depend on an individual's and group's concept of person.

Is person perceived within a dualistic framework, that is, body and soul, mind and body, or is the perception within the concept of unicity? Programs reflecting a dualistic concept are designed with an approach directed to each dualistic component, with some suggestion of synthesis, whereas programs reflecting the concept of unicity are designed with a single integrated approach.

Milhollan and Forisha (1972) identify two current diverse models of man— behavioristic and phenomenological—with which they feel individuals working with people need to be knowledgeable and aware of paradoxes.

> *The behavioristic orientation considers man to be a passive organism governed by stimuli supplied by the external environment. Man can be manipulated, that is, his behavior controlled through proper control of environmental stimuli.*
>
> *The phenomenological orientation considers man to be the source of all acts. Man is essentially free to make choices in each solution. The focal point of his freedom is human consciousness. Behavior is thus only the observable*

expressions and consequences of an essentially private, internal world of being (p.13).

The first model supports the concept of determinism and accepts the idea that a person's behavior is predictable. Frankl (1963) denies the concept of pan-determinism and believes that the greatest force in an individual's life is the search for meaning as it relates to the self at any point in time. He states, ". . . Man is not fully conditioned and determined; he determines himself whether to give in to conditions or stand up to them. In other words, Man is self determining" (p. 206). In reference to a person's predictability, he states, ". . . every human being has the freedom to change at any instant. Therefore we can predict his future only within the large frame of a statistical survey referring to a whole group; the individual personality, however, remains essentially unpredictable" (p. 20).

The two models certainly are not the only possible ones, but they are presented here to illustrate divergent concepts of the nature of person and his behavior; each would influence the type of behavioral outcome identified for a program of studies or a particular learning experience.

Exploration of the concept of person must include beliefs about an individual's response to stimuli in the internal and external environments. Stressors are inherent in all aspects of living, and questions need to be raised as to a person's ability to adapt in the search for balance in life. Behavioral responses to stimuli represent a multiple, complex interaction in which harmony and accord are sought in terms of the values and needs at any time period in the individual's life. Individuals have resiliency and can adapt to disharmony. Beliefs about their potential for as well as their approaches to coping with or altering the environment influence behaviors deemed appropriate for a program in the helping professions.

SOCIETAL GOALS AND TRENDS

The total spectrum of nursing, its practice, educational programs, research, and role within the health care system occurs within a rapidly changing macrosystem, society. The phenomenon of nursing must be studied within the context of that society in terms of present trends and future goals if its true meaning is to be understood. Since the lives of the students, faculty, and clients are closely interwoven in that society, practice and educational decisions are affected.

Knowledge about the society on a local, national, and international level is an essential element in preparing objectives for a program of study or a particular learning experience. Multiple forces, some conflicting, are in operation as the new century approaches. Of particular concern to nursing is the issue of allocation of finite financial resources within the present system of health care delivery which is failing to meet society's goal of health care for all. Moccia (1988) posits that the present "technocratic, fee-for-service health care system now lacks expertise or skill to meet the health care needs of a population that is increasingly aged, chronically ill, poor, and without access to reimbursed health services" (p. 30).

The maldistribution of money under such a system is resulting in support for expensive technologic acute care at the expense of money for prevention and long-term, chronic care. Fries (1986) sees the medical model of health care as inappropriate and urges all health care workers to adopt the goal of compression of morbidity. This concept calls for delaying the health problems associated with aging until later in life rather than in middle-life as is occurring now. Health care would entail placing greater emphasis on health education, decreasing health risk factors, and fostering preventive life-styles.

Because technocratic intervention in the course of a disease prolongs life, but not necessarily its quality, it raises serious ethical and moral questions for clients, society, families, and health professionals. The expense of many of these interventions, such as transplants, requires moral decisions as to who will receive their benefits. Ross (1984) warns that economic triage, the process whereby the selection of persons who can avail themselves of the advances in health care is based on economic resources, is already a reality.

Although the health care environment is directly related to the nursing profession, other social issues and trends are of equal significance. As 1990 begins, American society is being challenged about its failure to educate its citizens for the modern world. Issues center around who should pay for public education, what domains of knowledge and skills should be included in a program and how should the inequities of financial support between suburban communities and inner cities be addressed. Concern is also expressed about how the moral and ethical values of the society, particularly those espoused in the Bill of Rights, should be taught. Questions about higher education opportunities address who should attend, how financing should be achieved, and what domains of knowledge and expertise are needed by society.

Disintegration of society is seen on many fronts and calls upon innovative humanistic social solutions. Violence has become a way of life for many as instant gratification and its selection as a solution for perceived or real wrongs becomes the norm. Drugs are robbing our communities of their valuable resource, youth, and racism impedes free interchange among people on a human level. The resources to meet the basics of shelter and food are not allocated in sufficient amounts so that many are homeless.

World events are rapidly brought to our attention through a highly developed communication system. Cultural meanings, mores, and behaviors of many groups in the world are now made evident providing opportunity to increase our understanding of the human family. Power bases are shifting throughout the world as people seek more control of their lives, thus posing new problems and opportunities. As a result, professionals must refuse any form of parochial view of their field and be ready to adopt a world cosmopolitan view. Environmental destruction, poverty, violence, health deficits, and migration are merely several problems of world importance.

The issues and trends raised here are not inclusive but serve to increase faculty's understanding of the concerns which must be acknowledged in developing objectives. Other such concerns will be generated by individuals involved in program planning. These concerns are reality, the real world in which nurses are educated and function. They influence remarkably the goals and objectives and the knowledge context within which selected skills are developed. Education carried on in an insular manner contributes to a professional who is primarily technical rather than a professional who uses his or her skills within the context of the needs of society in any particular period of time.

PROFESSIONAL GOALS AND TRENDS

Nursing as a profession is being propelled at a rapid pace into conflicting currents of change within society, not only as a responder, but increasingly as an initiator and active participant. Empowerment of nursing in health matters is a proclaimed goal as nurses seek autonomy, an active decision-making role in the work place and the health care field, and control over the destiny of the profession. In the 1990s, nursing has multiple opportunities to impact on the larger health care system as a whole, which is also undergoing change. Are nurses ready to seize the opportunities and accept a role of social responsibility?

The perception of what nursing will be like in the next century will be a critical factor as nurse educators develop goals and objectives for programs of study. The 1990s already show trends, which if followed, will markedly alter the role of nursing in the delivery of health care within society. A value on the medical model "hi-tech care" places an even greater demand for nurses skilled in "hi-touch." Care as a critical element in nursing is being studied through research, and moral and ethical decision-making practices are receiving high priority. Advocacy, not only in client situations, but also in all levels of government relative to health matters has become an expected role of the profession.

Competency in use of power and its concomitment accountability is being assumed by nurses in the social, economic, political, and health care venues.

Movements within nursing itself are enabling it to assume a leading role in affecting the direction of some societal changes. Nursing's educational base for professional practitioners is comparable to that of other professionals with whom nurses associate. Several current practices suggest trends toward master's preparation for professionals; registered nurses from diploma and associate degree programs may opt to enter programs leading directly to a master degree in nursing when they return to school. Schools are now developing master in nursing or doctorate in nursing programs as entry preparation for graduates of colleges or universities with degrees in other fields. The doctorate degree, whether doctor of philosophy or doctor of nursing science, is now the terminal degree in nursing education accompanied by an increase in post-doctoral study. The schema of education in the profession provides for both technical and professional education with mobility possible through various levels as nurses change career goals and seek the necessary preparation.

Such educational advancement has been in concert with the growth in professional scholarship in nursing theory; research in nursing deepens our base of practice and nursing authors contribute to the literature of the field. Practice too has been altered as the new knowledge from research and experience is internalized. Nursing as a key participant in the movement for prevention of illness and promotion of health is proclaimed, but the current emphasis on the medical model of cure in society has deterred the movement from reaching its potential. Changes in community nursing practice are the result of a prospective system of payment for hospital service, based on diagnosis related groups (DRGs), which return patients to communities with therapeutic needs that were formerly the domain of nurses practicing in hospital and other inpatient settings.

At the same time, technologic advances have brought about an information society with significant implications for nursing. Computers are now integral parts of the health care delivery system and capable of organizing the multi-faceted data pertinent to agency function. Information systems are established in nursing departments, but often the linkage to other relevant departments is lacking. A linkage to the business office could facilitate nursing's desire to develop a system for costing out the nursing resource component of patient care. Computer systems that include protocols of care with data readily retrievable can expedite the planning process and facilitate more effective patient care management. Reilly and Oermann (1985) note the value of computers in nursing care in providing readily retrievable data not only relative to a particular client, but also types of clinical data that facilitate the identification of nursing knowledge, the selection of researchable questions, and precision in decision-making.

Nurses are recognized as a vital resource to society. The perceived shortage of nurses to meet the demands of health care agencies reinforces this belief. The shortage may be a function of greater breadth of career options in the field, misuse of nurses in agencies, or dissatisfaction with agency restrictions on practice as professionals. Whatever the cause, the present situation provides opportunities for nurses to compete more equitably for health care dollars, to receive appropriate compensation for services provided, and to assume more control over decisions which affect nursing.

Movements in nursing are occurring rapidly and often mean new directions. It behooves nursing educators to prepare individuals to practice within a society characterized by ambiguity rather than certainty where new problems cannot rely on past solutions. The goals and objectives must relate to the concept of nursing and its meaning within the larger society. The definition of nursing stated in the American Nurses' Association Social Policy Statement (1980) specifies "Nursing is the diagnosis and treatment of human responses to actual or real potential health problems" (p. 9). This definition accommodates varied clients whether they be an individual, a family, a group, or a community. As objectives are prepared in light of this definition, they must be stated in terms of the directions in which nursing is moving while still recognizing its rich heritage. The knowledge context in which these objectives are to be realized must also reflect trends. Donley (1984) identifies dimensions of knowledge as a "gestalt of technical, humanistic, and ethical knowledge" (p. 6). The gestalt represents the skill in using knowledge in clinical decisions, the philosophical knowledge essential for understanding the meaning of health, illness, life, death, and so forth, and the ethical knowledge to assess clinical decisions and social policies in terms of their rightness.

The objectives pertinent to nursing as it moves into the next century should reflect such competences as clinical judgment, reflective thinking, moral decision-making, caring and expert ministrations to clients, ability to work with ambiguity, collaboration, and use of power and its resultant accountability and skill in identifying problems and proposing appropriate strategies for solution. Of extreme importance is the ability to be a continuous learner.

NATURE OF THE LEARNER

Regardless of the educational endeavor, the learner is the focal point, for it is the learner's behavior that is to be developed in accord with stated goals. Since the program is designed for the student, participants in program development must be knowledgeable about the goals, values, interests, and learning style of the learner in addition to the usual demographic data about social, cultural, and academic background.

The kinds of data one seeks about the learner originate from beliefs about learners and reflect concepts about the nature of person. Is the learner to be controlled or is the learner to become a self-controlling individual with impulses and desires ordered by intelligence? Is the learner someone to whom things are done or someone who does things? What does research suggest about learner responses in the learning situation?

If educational programs are viewed within a developmental context, they start where the students are and direct them toward greater use of their potential. Therefore, knowledge of students at the point of entry into an educational experience is essential if behavioral objectives are to be realistic. It is important that instructors guard against projecting their own prejudicial or value connotations when interpreting data. The homogeneity of nursing students in terms of life style, social and economic background, educational experience, and values has given way to diversity as various ethnic, socioeconomic age groups enter nursing programs.

As nursing educational opportunities are made available to groups in our society that were previously disenfranchised from higher education, nursing has become an avenue of upward mobility for many individuals. For some, nursing provides the opportunity for career employment as the changing socioeconomic scene places limitations on employment possibilities in some career fields. For others, nursing is an opportunity for fulfillment of a desire for service to others. Motivations for entering nursing and for participating in programs of study beyond the basic preparation are varied and complex. The diversity of motivating forces in any group of nursing learners must be recognized by program planners.

Research about students within the context of learning has provided important data for faculty to use in assessing the student's potential and the response to learning experiences. Desired outcome behaviors of students can remain constant, but the learning experiences selected for students may vary. Paths to objective attainment are often many. In too many instances, teaching methodologies are proclaimed without due consideration of variations in student response to the methods, some of which may be dysfunctional.

Bloom (1982) believes that history of the student is the core of learning and is essential knowledge to predicting and recognizing the students' responses to any learning tasks. His research into entry behaviors, those required for a particular learning task or course, suggests that they are a key variable in accounting for the learning of students, and when not possessed by a group of students on an equitable basis they can account for up to one-half of the variance of achievement.

Rogers (1983) describes the efforts of a sixth grade teacher to institute a self-directed approach to classroom learning. Within a short time after its initiation, she noted that some students became frustrated and felt insecure without teacher direction. She instituted two groups in the class, self-directed and teacher-directed, with the intent of moving the students of the latter group toward self-direction at a slower pace. Readiness to engage in the "new" is a function of history and requisite entry behaviors.

Research in different ways individuals process information, the *how* of learning, not the *what*, has led to the identification of two major cognitive styles of learners: field-dependent and field-independent. Through the research of Witkin, Moore, Goodenough, and Cox (1977), differential characteristics in the processes of learning, perceiving, thinking, problem-solving and interactions with others, have been identified. Reilly and Oermann (1985) present a table which demonstrates the difference in characteristics. Field-independent learners are high in cognitive restructuring, and analytic and differential skills, are inner directed and motivated, but low in social response skills. Field-dependent students are more outer-directed, relying on social interactions and responses for motivation and approval, but are low in cognitive restructuring, analytic, and differential skills. Intelligence is not a concern here, but the way individuals process information. Thus, the selection of appropriate learning experience for meeting objectives is relevant. Field-independent learners respond most favorably to independent experiences which stimulate analytic skills with emphasis on lecture and discovery, while field-dependent students respond best to group interaction strategies with the responsibility shared by instructor and learner.

Research by Milton, Pollio, and Eison (1986) presents another variant among students that, although acknowledged tacitly in practice, is seldom expressed in the literature. That variant pertains to the role that grades assume as motivators for learning. Two major classifications of students were identified, high-learning orientation and high grade-orientation, and characteristic responses toward the learning situation for each group were evident. Each group was subdivided:

1. High learning-orientation/high grade-orientation
   (High LO/High GO)

2. High learning-orientation/low grade-orientation
   (High LO/Low GO)

3. Low learning-orientation/high grade-orientation
   (Low LO/High GO)

4. Low learning-orientation/low grade-orientation
   (Low LO/Low GO)

In general, high learning-orientation represents inner locus of control, motivation toward pursuit of educational enrichment and personal growth, greater abstract reasoning, higher levels of sensitivity, and low tension. These learners generally are intellectually and emotionally able, willing, and interested. High grade-orientation represents outer locus of control, with all aspects of the educational experience viewed in terms of their effect on grades. These learners exhibit a high degree of tension and endure self-pressure to do the right thing and act in conventional ways. Their study habits tend to be poor, and they exhibit a concrete approach to learning tasks. Knowledge about the learning/grade orientation of students enables instructors to select strategies which maximize the learner's potential for attainment of the desired objectives.

The illustrations presented here are not meant to be inclusive, but they do suggest that responses to learning experiences are varied and often depend on the resources, past practices, and motivations of the learner. Open-ended objectives are appropriate for they state the desired behavioral outcome, but do not denote the teaching strategies to be used. The instructor who truly believes that learning is a transformational process recognizes that in any learning situation the ability to identify the student's proclivity and potential for engaging in the process is fundamental to the selection of the experience. For instance, nursing practice requires objectives related to cognitive skills of analysis (field-independent) and personal interaction skills (field-dependent). The clinical instructor, using knowledge of cognitive styles, chooses experiences which foster the preference of each group while devising strategies for developing opposite skills. The goal of meeting both behaviors for each group is constant; the means by which the behaviors are developed varies according to the learning style of the learner.

CONCEPT OF THE TEACHING-LEARNING PROCESS

Instructional decisions made by teachers are numerous: nature of knowledge to be learned, objectives most relevant and attainable for a particular learner or group of learners, teaching strategies which facilitate achievement of objective, sequencing of knowledge and experiences, formative evaluation to identify cues from learner behavior, and summative evaluation of objective behavior outcomes, yet all this also accommodating goal-free learning. This basis of such decisions must be rooted in theory and fundamental values reflective of the integrity and worth of each student. It is essential that each teacher formulate a philosophy of education and a conceptual framework of the teaching-learning dynamic from which to make decisions. This framework is descriptive rather than predictive.

There are numerous theories of learning based on assumptions about the nature of person and the nature of knowledge which explain the process by which learning occurs. There is no one generally accepted theory. Likewise, there is no real theory of instruction which is predictive, but, as Bruner (1966) says, "a body of maxims to guide decisions" (p. 31). Efforts are underway to develop such a theory as exemplified by Bloom (1982) in his research of the relationship among cognitive entry characteristics, affective entry characteristics, and quality of instruction provided.

A conceptual framework must have consistency between beliefs about learning and beliefs about teaching because of the nature of their interrelationship. A framework may be derived from one particular theory of learning or may be eclectic composed of compatible elements from several theories. Two major classifications of learning theories exist: *natural science* represented by theories of association, conditioning, and behaviorism, and *human science* represented by theories of gestalt, cognitive field, social learning, humanism, and phenomenology. Both groups accept the notion that the outcome of learning is a change in behavior as the result of experience. The experience variable is essential to differentiate behavior change from learning from that associated with maturation or change in body structure or function.

The classifications just noted are derived from two distinct perceptions about the nature of person (man). Milhollan and Forisha (1972) describe these two differing theories in reference to the concept for a science basis for each.

Behaviorism. The laws that govern man are primarily the same as the universal laws that govern all natural phenomena. Therefore, the scientific method, as evolved by the physical sciences, is appropriate as well for the study of the human organism.

Phenomenology. Only a science of man which begins with experience, as it is immediately given in this world of being, can ever be adequate for a study of the human organism (p. 13).

Behaviorism as espoused by Skinner (1972) is the most frequent natural science theory in current usage. Learning is passive, mechanistic, deterministic, additive, and predictive—given a stimulus, one can predict behavior pattern and visa versa. All complexities of mental life can be reduced to small sensory experiences so that if the simple is known, the complex can be predicted. Concern with the internal or central processes of the mind is minimal, for emphasis is placed on observable stimulus and response. Reinforcement of a positive response which itself becomes a stimulus and increases the probability of a further response is a key concept in this theory. Teaching within this theory is directed toward controlling all contingencies in the learning situation so as to reinforce positive stimuli and strengthen subsequent behavior.

Human science theories of learning describe learning as active, holistic, unpredictable, goal-directed, integrated, and experiential. Learning is an individual process which emphasizes "meanings, principles and relationships among phenomena and is concerned with perception, insight and cognitive structure formation" (Reilly & Oermann, 1985, p. 29). Cognitive field theory stresses the role of cognitive disequilibrium as a stimulus for learning which calls upon critical thinking and problem solving for solution. Learning occurs through a change in the perception of the problem resulting in new insights or change in old ones. New learning becomes integrated into the learner's psychological field through the process of restructuring.

Phenomenological theory as described by Rogers (1983) stresses the role of experiencing in learning and the involvement of the total learner. Motivation arises from within the learner for those experiences which are significant for the learner's perceived needs for self-actualization. Rogers identifies five characteristics of this type of learning: "personal involvement, self-initiated, pervasive, evaluated by the learner, and its essence is meaning" (p. 5).

Both theories of learning are included in the category of human science for they support the notion of the psychological field of the individual and behavior as a function of that field at any given time. Internal locus of control, the significance of experience, the total involvement of the learner in interaction with the environment, and the cognitive processes of problem identification, insight formulation, search for meaning, and problem resolution are common concepts here.

Teaching within the context of theories of human science is a facilitating rather than a controlling process as found in natural science theories. It involves a transformation whereby the perceptual fields of teacher and learner are shared toward a goal-directed encounter with new experiences. It occurs within a climate of trust, authenticity, and caring where learners are supported as they enter into learning experiences which may involve risk and new use of self. It fosters the development of the self-directed learner skilled in use of resources. Teaching, like the nursing process, is diagnostic and interventive whereby data about students and cues from formative evaluation of learner behavior are used in individualizing the learner's instruction to the learning needs (Reilly & Oermann, 1985).

Because nursing is a humanistic, caring, scientifically-based practice discipline, learning theories from the human sciences classification are the most appropriate. Their emphasis on experiential learning and problem-solving are particularly relevant, since these two processes dominate the practice experience.

Experiences must be examined within the total context of education and the purposes to be met. Learner involvement is the constant variable noted by theorists in this science domain. James (1958), the renowned educational philosopher, feels that the greatest maxim which the teacher must hold is, "No reception without reaction—no impression without correlative expression" (p. 35). Tyler (1950) describes learning experiences as "the interaction between learner and the external conditions in the environment to which he can react. Learning takes place through the active behavior of the student; it is what *he* does that he learns, not what the teacher does" (p. 41). Dewey (1963) defines two characteristics of assuring that a learning experience is an educative one:

Continuity—takes something from those which have gone before and modifies in some way the qualities of those who come after. Continuity means continued growth.

Interaction—the experience is what it is because of the transaction taking place between an individual and what, at that time, constitutes own environment (pp. 33–34).

Schön (1990), in stressing the need for professionals to develop reflection in practice, refers to the artistry of the teacher, a coach expert in the process of guidance. Schön perceives clinical practice experience to be of high interpersonal intensity. Professional artistry refers to the kind of competence displayed by practitioners in unique, uncertain, and conflicting situations which is often in the realm of tacit knowledge (Schön, 1990). Teacher artistry is particularly relevant to the teacher's role as preceptor. Rogers (1983) perceives learning as, "Significant learning combines the logical and the intuitive, the intellect *and* the feelings, the concept *and* the experience, the idea *and* the meaning" (p. 20).

Much experiential learning experience involves problem-solving, focusing on the student's ability to seek meaning and order. Problem-solving experiences not only contribute to the student competency in meeting client needs, they also prepare students for practice in an ambiguous society where varied and often conflicting choices are required. Perspectives for alternative decisions and actions are developed and the students master the skill of learning how to learn so that a questioning posture is established for evaluating new and continuing practices, knowledges, and trends.

Are human science theories and the preparation of objectives compatible? It is the thesis of the authors that a conceptual framework of the teaching-learning processes derived from such theories provides a firm basis for preparation of objectives, provided that they are open-ended, reflective of reality, and stated at the appropriate level of student development.

PHILOSOPHY AND PURPOSE OF
AGENCY OFFERING THE PROGRAM

A program of studies operates within the framework of a specific agency which has its own social and educational philosophy. As part of that agency's system, the educational program must have objectives consistent with the expressed philosophy and purpose of that agency. Tyler (1950) perceives the educational and social philosophy of a school as a screen for selecting objectives most salient to the institution's beliefs and values. Behaviors inconsistent with the philosophy are discarded.

The same concept applies to staff development programs in health agencies. The agency's philosophy of nursing practice and its expressed commitment to staff development for its practitioners serve as a guide for formulating objectives for that program.

When a conflict occurs between the desire for attainment of a particular behavioral objective and the agency need to implement a philosophy not supportive of this behavior, the solution must be found in either changing the philosophy or discarding the objective. Faculty may want to express behavioral objectives in the higher cognitive skills, but if the philosophy of the school supports open admission, levels of behaviors must be geared to the highest level most students can achieve.

Thus, in the process of developing objectives, one must identify behaviors suggested by the philosophy of the agency and aim toward developing them in the program.

MODELS OF NURSING

Program developers in a profession refer to their theory of practice to aid them in identifying appropriate behaviors. This theory serves to focus the goals of the practice, to define its boundaries or parameters, and to describe its nature in relation to the clients served, the types of problems with which it is concerned, its methodology, and the value base upon which it rests.

Nursing as a science and practice discipline requires a theory of nursing practice. Argyris and Schön (1974) define a theory of practice:

A theory of practice consists of a set of interrelated theories of action that specify for the situations of the practice, the actions that will, under relevant assumptions, yield intended consequences. Theories of practice usually contain theories of intervention, that is, theories of action aimed at enhancing effectiveness; these may be differentiated according to roles in which intervention is attempted —for example, counseling and teaching (p. 16).

A theory of practice is essential for directing the endeavors of a profession. Without a theory base, a practice is subject to inconsistency, irrationality, and unpredictability as it becomes self-serving. These characteristics result primarily because its derivation is from intuition, imitation, or a professional mystique that surrounds some of its "successful" members rather than from a theoretical basis.

The practice theory then becomes the root of the profession which serves its practitioners, its educators, and its researchers. It is the *What*.

Nursing theory is evolving as research in nursing practice generates the new knowledge necessary to make the phenomena of nursing ever more explicit. Such evolution is essential if nursing is to have its own science, a critical criterion for any profession.

During the past few decades, various conceptual models and theories have been proposed, examined, refined, and continuously subject to critical analysis in nursing. Four concerns of nursing—person, environment, health, and nursing—are integral parts of all notions of nursing theory; it is the approach to these concerns and their description within the concept of nursing that varies. Of the recently proposed models and theories postulated and researched, some may be of value to particular faculty who are developing conceptual model curriculum for their programs. The samples of models and theories presented below are inclusive of course:

Roy's Adaptation Model (Roy & Roberts, 1981) views persons as adaptive systems in constant interaction with the environment.

Orem's Self-Care Model (Orem, 1985) is built upon the notion of a person's self-care needs and the capabilities to meet these needs.

Rogers' Theory of Unitary Human Beings (Rogers, 1970) views persons as whole, integrated entities, not in terms of parts.

King's General Systems Model (King, 1989) emphasizes the interactions of persons and the environment, particularly in relation to interpersonal processes involved between caregiver and carerecipient.

Neuman's General Systems Model (Neuman, 1989) relates to the ability of the client system to cope with stressors in the environment.

Watson's Theory of Human Caring (Watson, 1985) addresses the moral and ethical dimensions of nursing.

Leininger's Theory of Culture Care Diversity and Universality (Leininger, 1988) postulates care as the essence of nursing with cultural variability in expression.

Benner's Caring Model (Benner & Wrubel, 1989) relates the phenomenon of caring to stress management in health and illness.

The reader is urged to go to the direct sources of these various theories and models in preparation for developing a conceptual framework for curriculum.

Conceptual models are not theoretical models. Reilly (1975) differentiates between the two. A conceptual model (framework) provides a perspective, a way of looking at nursing. It is a representation of reality since it is derived from and pertains to reality, but it does not constitute reality. A theoretical model (framework) on the other hand does constitute reality since it has a scientifically accepted basis.

A conceptual model for a framework of a nursing program provides a unified approach to ordering objectives, content, course selection and placement, learning experiences, and evaluation (Reilly, 1975). Fawcett (1988) sees a model as a guideline for nursing practice in assisting the clinician in focusing on client observations, clinical decision-making, and evaluation for outcome. Gordon (1982) considers a model as essential for determining a nursing diagnosis for it provides guidelines for clinical data gathering, interpretation and meaning.

Presently, no one conceptual model or theory is acknowledged as universal. That is as it should be at this time in theory development. Faculty may select a particular theory or model of nursing as a basis for the curriculum framework, or may choose to design an eclectic framework from various theories. Whatever the decision, it must be a faculty decision, for the maintenance of the integrity of the model is a function of the instructors charged with its implementation. Once a model is selected, objectives are written in accord with the direction provided by the model and the program of studies is developed and implemented accordingly, inclusive of evaluation of outcomes compatible with the model.

SUMMARY

Derivation of the substance of objectives involves carefully exploring at least seven areas: the nature of person, societal goals and trends, professional goals and trends, the nature of the learner, the concept of the teaching–learning process, philosophy and goals of the agency, and models of nursing.

Examination of these seven areas with identification of their meanings and implications is essential for developing objectives that are relevant to nursing, its discipline, its practice and its role within the health care system and pertinent to the needs of the learner during the educational process. Content of learning is not the critical factor, but rather it is the behavior of the learners as they participate in the experiences and achieve the ultimate goal.

Nursing is a complex, multifaceted profession drawn from the human rather than the natural sciences for its basis. So too should the human science base be used for the teaching of that discipline. Objectives must reflect that dynamic in their expression.

Development of conceptual models and theories of nursing is advancing rapidly as research proceeds at a rigorous pace. The current theories and models afford an excellent opportunity for faculty to devise a nursing-driven conceptual framework curriculum.

REFERENCES

American Nurses' Association. (1980). *Nursing: A social policy statement.* Kansas City: The Author.

Argyris, C., & Schön, D. (1974). *Theory in practice: Increasing professional effectiveness.* San Francisco: Jossey-Bass.

Benner, P., & Wrubel, J. (1989). *The primacy of caring: Stress and coping in health and illness.* Menlo Park, CA: Addison-Wesley.

Bloom, B. S. (1982). *Human characteristics and school learning.* New York: McGraw-Hill.

Bruner, J. S. (1966). *Toward a theory of instruction.* Cambridge: Belknap Press of Harvard University Press.

Chickering, A. W. (1969). *Education and identity.* San Francisco: Jossey-Bass.

Dewey, J. (1963). *Experience in education.* New York: Collin Books.

Donley, R., Sr. (1984). Nursing: 2000, an essay. *Image, 16*(1), 4–6.

Fawcett, J. (1988). *Analysis and evaluation of conceptual models of nursing* (2nd ed.). Philadelphia: F.A. Davis.

Frankl, V. (1963). *Man's search for meaning.* New York: Washington Square Press.

Fries, J. F. (1986). The future of disease and treatment. *Journal of Professional Nursing, 2*(1), 10–18.

Gordon, M. (1982). *Nursing diagnosis: Process and application.* New York: McGraw-Hill.

James, W. (1958). *Talks to teachers.* New York: W.W. Norton Co.

King, I. (1989). King's general systems framework and theory. In J. Riehl-Sisca (Ed.), *Conceptual models for nursing practice* (pp. 149–158). Norwalk, CT: Appleton & Lange.

Leininger, M. (1988). Leininger's theory of nursing: Cultural care diversity and universality. *Nursing Science Quarterly, 1*(4), 152–160.

Milhollan, F., & Forisha, B. (1972). *From Skinner to Rogers*. Lincoln, NE: Professional Educators.

Milton, O., Pollio, H., & Eisen, J. (1986). *Making sense of college grades*. San Francisco: Jossey-Bass.

Moccia, P. (1988). At the faultline: Social activism and caring. *Nursing Outlook, 36*(1), 30–33.

Neuman, R. (1989). *The Neuman system model* (2nd ed.). Norwalk, CT: Appleton-Century-Crofts.

Orem, D. (1985). *Nursing concepts of practice* (3rd ed.). New York: McGraw-Hill.

Reilly, D. (1975). Why a conceptual framework? *Nursing Outlook. 23*(9), 566–569.

Reilly, D., & Oermann, M. (1985). *The clinical field: Its use in nursing education*. Norwalk, CT: Appleton-Century-Crofts.

Rogers, C. (1983). *Freedom to learn for the 1980's*. Columbus: Charles Merrill.

Rogers, M. (1970). *An introduction to the theoretical basis of nursing*. Philadelphia: F.A. Davis.

Ross, V. (1984). The right to die debate. *World Press Review*, pp. 32–34.

Roy, D., & Roberts, S. (1981). *Theory construction in nursing: An adaptation model*. Englewood Cliffs, NJ: Prentice-Hall.

Schön, D. A. (1990). *Educating the reflective practitioner*. San Francisco: Jossey-Bass.

Skinner, B. (1972). *Beyond freedom and dignity*. New York: Random House.

Tyler, R. (1950). *Basic principles of curriculum and instruction*. Chicago: University of Chicago.

Watson, J. (1985). *Nursing: Human science and human care*. Norwalk, CT: Appleton-Century-Crofts.

Witkin, H., Moore, C., Goodenough, D., & Cox, P. (1977). Field-dependent and field-independent cognitive styles and their educational implications. *Review of Educational Research, 47*, 1–64.

RECOMMENDED READINGS

Aaronsen, L. (1985). A challenge for nursing: Gaining recognition as a profession distinct from medicine. *Nursing Outlook, 37*(4), 274–275.

American Association of Colleges of Nursing. (1986). *Essentials of college and university education for nursing*. Washington, DC: The Author.

Andrews, H., & Roy, C., Sr. (1986). *Essentials of the Roy adaptation model*. Norwalk, CT: Appleton-Century-Crofts.

Barnum, B. (1987). Nursing: Now, then, and maybe again. *Nursing Outlook, 35*(5), 219–221.

Barrett, E. (Ed.). (1990). *Visions of Rogers' science-based nursing*. New York: National League for Nursing.

Benner, P. (1984). *From novice to expert: Excellence and power in clinical practice.* Menlo Park, CA: Addison-Wesley.

Bevis, E., & Watson, J. (1989). *Toward a caring curriculum: A new pedagogy for nursing.* New York: National League for Nursing.

Bigge, M. (1976). *Learning theories for teachers* (3rd ed.). New York: Harper & Row.

Booth, R. (1985). Financing mechanism for health care: Impact on nursing services. *Journal of Professional Nursing, 1*(1), 34–40.

Chin, P. (1989). Nursing patterns of knowing and feminist thought. *Nursing and Health Care, 10*(2), 71–75.

Clayton, G., & Murray, J. (1989). Faculty-student relationships: Catalytic connection. In National League for Nursing, *Curriculum revolution: Reconceptualizing nursing education* (pp. 43–53). New York: National League for Nursing.

Crowley, M. (1989). Feminist pedagogy: Nurturing the ethical ideal. *Advance in Nursing Science, 11*(3), 53–61.

De Back, V. (1987). National Commission on nursing implementation project. *Journal of Professional Nursing, 3*(4), 226–229.

Detner, S. (1986). The future of health care delivery system and settings. *Journal of Professional Nursing, 2*(1), 20–27.

Diers, D. (1987). When college grads choose nursing. *American Journal of Nursing, 87*(12), 1631–1637.

Donely, R., Sr. (1988). Building nursing's platform for the long-term care debate. *Nursing & Health Care, 9*(6), 303–305.

Downes, F. (1988). Doctoral education: Our claim to the future. *Nursing Outlook, 36*(1), 18–20.

Eble, K. (1973). *Professors as teachers.* San Francisco: Jossey-Bass.

Eble, K. (1988). *The craft of teaching* (2nd ed.). San Francisco: Jossey-Bass.

Forni, P. (1987). Nursing's diverse master's programs: The state of the art. *Nursing & Health Care, 8*(2), 71–75.

Forni, P., & Welch, M. (1987). The professional vs. the academic model: A dilemma for nursing education. *Journal of Professional Nursing, 3*(5), 291–297.

Fry, S. (1988). The ethics of caring: Can it survive in nursing? *Nursing Outlook, 36*(1), 45.

Hanchett, E. (1988). *Nursing frameworks and community as client: Bridging the gap.* Norwalk, CT: Appleton & Lange.

Harrington, C. (1988). A policy agenda for nursing shortage. *Nursing Outlook, 36*(3), 118–119.

Hedin, B. (1989). Expert clinical teaching. In National League for Nursing, *Curriculum revolution: Reconceptualizing nursing education* (pp. 71–89). New York: National League for Nursing.

Holleran, C. (1988). Nursing beyond national borders. *Nursing Outlook, 36*(2), 72–75.

Institute of Medicine. (1983). *Nursing and nursing education: Public policies and private actions.* Washington, DC: National Academy Press.

Johnson, J. (1987). Essentials for collegiate and university education for professional nursing. *Journal of Professional Nursing, 3*(4), 207–213.

Kidd, P., & Morrison, E. (1988). The progression of knowledge in nursing: A search for meaning. *Image, 20*(4), 222–224.

Maglacos, A. (1988). Health for all: Nursing's role. *Nursing Outlook, 36*(2), 66–71.

Martin, S. (1990). Research on differences between baccalaureate and associate degree nurses. In C. Clayton & P. Baj (Eds.), *Review of research in nursing education* (Vol. III, pp. 109–146). New York: National League for Nursing.

McNerney, A. (1988). Nursing's vision in a competitive environment. *Nursing Outlook, 36*(3), 126–129.

Meyers, C. (1986). *Teaching students to think critically.* San Francisco: Jossey-Bass.

Miller, M., & Malcolm, N. (1990). Critical thinking in the nursing curriculum. *Nursing & Health Care, 11*(2), 67–73.

Milo, N. (1985). Telematics in future of health care delivery. *Journal of Professional Nursing, 2*(1), 39–50.

Mitchell, C. (1988). One view of the future non-traditional education as the norm. *Nursing & Health Care, 9*(4), 187–190.

Oermann, M. H. (1990). Research on teaching methods. In C. Clayton & P. Baj (Eds.), *Review of research in nursing education* (Vol. III, pp. 1–32). New York: National League for Nursing.

Orlando, T., & Dugan, A. (1989). Independent and dependent paths: The fundamental issues for the nursing profession. *Nursing & Health Care, 10*(2), 77–80.

Rogers, M. (1985). The nature and characteristics of professional education for nursing. *Journal of Professional Nursing, 1*(6), 381–383.

Schein, E. (1972). *Professional education: Some new directions.* New York: McGraw-Hill.

Scholfeldt, R. (1987). Resolution of issues: An imperative for creating nursing's future. *Journal of Professional Nursing, 3*(3), 136–142.

Schön, D. (1983). *The reflective practitioner.* New York: Basic Books.

Stevenson, J., & Tripp-Reimer, T. (Eds.). (1990). *Knowledge about care and caring: State of the art and future developments.* Kansas City: American Academy of Nursing.

Tanner, C. A., & Lindemann, C. A. (1987). Research in nursing education: Assumptions and priorities. *Journal of Nursing Education, 26*(2), 50–59.

Tiessen, J. B. (1987). Critical thinking and selected correlates among baccalaureate nursing students. *Journal of Professional Nursing, 3*(2), 118–123.

Williams, C. (Ed.). (1983). *Image making in nursing.* Kansas City: American Nurses' Association.

Zwolski, K. (1989). Professional nursing in a technical system. *Image, 21*(4), 238–242.

3

Development of Behavioral Objectives

Once the substance of the objectives has been identified through exploration of the seven areas discussed in the previous chapter and after synthesis of their common elements, program developers write behavioral objectives that truly communicate the intent of the planners. Objectives are tools that guide all activities of the program designers and participants in the educational endeavor. Formulation of these objectives represents the conscious choice of the planners and is expressed in terms that are clear to all who are involved in implementation.

Behavioral objectives are expressed in relation to students, not teachers. The educational endeavor is geared toward change in the learner's behavior and it is this change that is to be evaluated. The real purpose is not to assay what the teacher does. That is not to say that the teacher's behavior is not also subject to change during this academic endeavor and indeed, if a transformative interaction is occurring, the teacher also will be a learner. Teachers might set up behavioral objectives for themselves as a tool for self-evaluation. However, program developers devise behavioral objectives addressed to those changes indicated for the learner.

There are two dimensions to the preparation of behavioral objectives. One relates to the technique of writing objectives and will be discussed in this chapter. The second is concerned with ordering behaviors according to the complexity of each. This latter will be developed in subsequent chapters dealing with the concept of taxonomy.

COMPONENTS OF A BEHAVIORAL OBJECTIVE

The development of behavioral objectives represents a very inexact field of endeavor and, indeed, the literature on this subject reflects various points of view. It is important to recognize that there are several formulas for writing objectives, and that the use intended for behavioral objectives determines the choice of an appropriate formula. Review of the literature suggests two major classifications for behavioral objectives—specific and general. The prescription for each of these types will be presented and their meaning and use discussed.

Specific Behavioral Objectives

The prescription for this type of objective was proposed by behaviorists and other natural science educators, particularly in response to the necessity for behavioral objective specificity in program planning.

In general there are four elements in the objective:

1. Description of the learner.
2. Description of the behavior the learner will exhibit to demonstrate that competence has been attained.
3. Description of conditions under which the learner will demonstrate competence. The description notes specific restrictions imposed.
4. Statement of standard of performance expected to indicate excellence.

EXAMPLE: Given a slide tape in which a man and a woman read Rod McKuen's poem, "Knowing When to Leave," the nursing student will identify, in writing, the difference in communication between men and women in terms of pitch, voice, enunciation, and facial expressions.

ANALYSIS OF THE BEHAVIORAL OBJECTIVE

1. Description of the learner	Nursing student
2. Description of the behavior	Identify in writing communication differences between men and women.
3. Description of conditions	Given a slide tape of a woman and man reading the Rod McKuen poem, "Knowing When to Leave."

4. Statement of standard
Four differences must be discussed: pitch, voice, enunciation, facial expression.

General Behavioral Objectives

The prescription was suggested by Tyler (1950) and others. Kibler, Barker, and Miles (1970) call this type of objective informational. Basically there are three elements in this type of behavioral objective.

1. Description of the learner.
2. Statement of the kind of behavior the learner will exhibit to demonstrate competence has been attained.
3. Statement of the kind of content to which behavior relates. (Kibler et al. combine 2 and 3.)

EXAMPLE: The nursing student distinguishes differences between male and female patterns of communication.

ANALYSIS OF THE BEHAVIORAL OBJECTIVE

1. Description of the learner   Nursing student
2. Description of the behavior   Distinguish differences
3. Statement of content   Male and female patterns of communication

GENERALITY VS. SPECIFICITY

The two approaches to writing behavioral objectives have similarities and differences. In essence, they are similar in two fundamental aspects: they agree that the learner must be specified, and they agree that the objective must be expressed in terms of behavior. The difference occurs in the desirability of including specific information about conditions of learning and criteria for performance acceptance. Both types of objectives can be accommodated in a program of studies, the choice, however, reflects the knowledge of their intent and the assumptions underlying their preparation.

Specific objectives with learning contingencies incorporated within the statement are close-ended and provide little flexibility for the teacher and learner during the learning experience. Previous discussions note that these behavioral objectives are based on the assumptions of the natural science school of thought, especially behaviorism. Learning within this context is perceived to be mechanistic, additive, and manipulative. The complexity of the learning dynamic in many fields of study such as nursing is antithetical to the use of such a rigid, prescriptive, and predictive approach to the statement of outcomes.

Specificity of behavioral objectives for a program of studies raises many concerns for program planners. The incorporation of a specific evaluation strategy with criteria negate the notion that individuals may vary in the manner in which they express outcomes, thus suggesting a variety of strategies as more appropriate. Unfortunately, many individuals equate the term *evaluation* with the term *testing*. Therefore, when the evaluation is specified in the statement, a testing perspective enters the teaching–learning situation. Durbach, Goodall, and Wilkinson (1987) reflect this perspective in stating that one of the indices for not using objectives in patient teaching is when there is no intent to test patients to see if they have learned. Inherent in teaching is evaluation, a continuous formative process as the teaching proceeds, to ascertain learners' responses. The responses do not need to be tested. However, objectives do need to be evaluated, for the teacher is accountable. The rationale for objectives is unrelated to the intent of testing; their role is direction setting for learning experience.

Generality as a characteristic format for writing objectives is more compatible with the dynamic of learning, for it provides for individual differences in the process. A general format is based on the assumptions derived from human science schools of thought where learning is perceived to be an active, involved experiential process. These objectives are open-ended. They clarify expected outcome, but leave students and faculty free to determine the path to the objective and the approach to evaluation. This enables the teaching–learning process to become personal, human, and facilitating, since the learner's needs, interests, and capabilities can be considered in reaching the expressed outcome. Since all the "givens" are not provided, the creative potentials of the teacher and learner are aroused and have opportunity for development. Furthermore, since the focus of participants is not limited, all are able to identify and capitalize on collateral learnings that often occur as well.

The view of generality is expressed by several theorists. Tyler (1950) supports the concept of generality when he states, "I tend to view objectives as general modes of reaction to be developed, rather than specific habits to be acquired" (p. 28). He further states, "So far as behavioral aspect of objectives is concerned, the problem of generality and specificity is one of obtaining the level of generality desired and what is in harmony with what we know about the psychology of learning" (p. 37).

Bloom (1956) believes that specifics are best learned in relation to general abstractions.

> *When learning takes place in this way, it is possible for an individual who remembers the generalization to proceed relatively easily to some specifics subsumed under generalization. On the other hand, generalization or abstraction are relatively difficult to learn unless they are related to appropriate concrete phenomenon (pp. 35–36).*

Because the general format objective is open-ended, it lends itself to use with higher cognitive skills, and especially where the experiential component of learning is critical as participants grasp for meaning and order in the phenomena they are dealing with. Evaluation, rather than being prescribed by objectives, respects the personal involvement of the learner and teacher in the problem-solving process so that both process and outcome are addressed. Higher levels of learning cannot be confined by the parameters of controlled contingencies in the situation; they must develop in a free, goal-directed environment where all potentials and possibilities can be maximized for learning. The world of nursing is not controlled, it is ambiguous and everchanging and thus requires skills of analysis, critical thinking, judgment, and readiness to develop new approaches to issues and problems in practice and society.

USE OF SPECIFIC AND GENERAL BEHAVIORS

From previous discussions, it is apparent that a different premise underlies each type of behavioral objective, general and specific, and that uses for each type vary.

The specific format for writing behavioral objectives has limited use; although efforts to use it have been varied and extensive since it was first proposed. In linear programmed instruction, the specificity may be an asset by focusing the process on step by step learning, characteristic of the additive learning assumption in behaviorism and building on specific behaviors for reinforcement. The format may also be used with a sharply delimited learning experience, especially where a low level skill is the outcome and consistency in performance is important (e.g., teaching a patient to test urine).

The general objective format is most appropriate for the statement of outcomes of a program or learning experience. Objectives of this type can be limited to a reasonable number since their scope is broader. Their openness encourages instructors to be more creative in their teaching and accommodate variations of behavior found in students.

Objectives in this general format are particularly important in a professional field where knowledge is not an accumulation of specific parts, but rather an integrated whole designated as concepts and theories. Nurses do not amass items of information; they use synthesized bodies of knowledge in their role as practitioners. Dewey (1961) emphasizes the significance of knowledge utilization in his definition of knowledge, "perception of the connections of an object which determine its applicability in a given situation" (p. 340). He considers knowledge to be "such a network on interconnections that any past experience would offer a point of advantage from which to get at the problem presented in a new experience" (p. 340). Whitehead (1958) is well known for his warning about inert ideas, for it is their utilization that is meaningful.

Behavioral objectives which foster creative utilization of ideas and knowledge are stated in general terms in accord with a taxonomy in the relevant domain of learning, cognitive, psychomotor, or affective. This process is described in the following chapter. It is a significant process to assure that objectives will be relevant, at the appropriate level of complexity and stated throughout the program of studies as directional progress goals.

POINTS IN WRITING BEHAVIORAL OBJECTIVES

Many books and articles have dealt with the technique for writing behavioral objectives. References included at the end of this chapter contain suggestions for sources this writer found helpful. A few major points about technique are, however, germane. In principle, objectives should be written clearly, concisely, and in the vernacular of the learner.

Behavioral Terms

The critical aspect of any behavioral objective is the word selected to indicate expected behavior from an educational experience. As considered by some, a behavioral term must be observable and measurable. Behavior generally is construed to be any action of an individual that can be seen, felt, or heard by another person. A concept of action implies psychomotor involvement. Kibler et al. (1970) warn us about overemphasizing the action component of objectives when they state, "Cognitive and affective objectives are concerned with characteristics of thinking and feeling which are themselves not directly observable. States of affection and acts of cognition are *inferred* from psychomotor acts." As an illustration, they add: "We do not see a person analyze a poem; we see or hear a report of his analysis" (p. 321). Thus the significant characteristic of the behavioral term is its measurability.

Some words commonly found in objectives, however, imply no action. The terms *understanding, knowledge,* and *appreciation* are nonactive and provide no direction for program development or qualitative assessment. Indeed, the term *understanding* can represent any of a wide range of cognitive processes, from simple to complex. Since the major function of behavioral objectives is communication, the terms used must be defined by the individuals concerned so that all interpret the words similarly and use them consistently with the same intent. A list of suggested action verbs appropriate for each level of the taxonomy for the three domains of learning is provided in Chapter 4.

One Behavior Per Objective

A behavioral objective expresses the intended outcome, not outcomes, of a learning experience and must be amenable to credentialing. One pattern of writing behavioral objectives frequently encountered shows that two or more behaviors have been included in one objective. This practice makes it difficult to evaluate the outcome, for the learner may attain one behavior but not the others. For example, the following behavioral objective includes two cognitive behaviors:

> *The nursing student identifies and analyzes phenomena in the patient's environment that influence the patient's ability to adapt to the limitations imposed by his or her illness.*

Two behaviors are involved here: *identifies* and *analyzes.* A student may indeed identify phenomena but not be able to analyze them in relation to their influence on the patient's adaptive response. Actually, if the behavioral objective stated the one behavior, *analyze,* it would be sufficient because identification of phenomena is an integral part of the analytic process.

Exclusion of Methodology in Statement

Another pitfall for developers of behavioral objectives is the tendency to include methodology in the statement of the objective. This practice places a severe limitation on the learner as well as the evaluator, for it states that there is only one way the student can learn a particular behavior and it permits the evaluator to assess that student's competency only in terms of the method specified. For example, the following behavioral objective includes a methodology restriction:

The nursing student demonstrates collaborative skills through maintenance of effective interpersonal interactions.

This behavior as stated suggests that only one dimension of collaborative skill is emphasized: maintaining effective interpersonal interactions. Furthermore, the evaluator's assessment is restricted to competence in collaborative skills according to this one criterion. It ignores many other criteria, such as the learner's assessment of the problem under discussion, problem-solving ability, and knowledge of nursing's particular contribution to the solution of the problem.

Another method may be injected into a statement of a behavioral objective. This method is the instructional procedure used to help the student attain the behavior. The following illustration includes a methodology, suggesting that a student's learning can be attained and validated only in terms of one procedure.

The nursing student develops through group discussion an awareness of the interrelationship between one's values and one's response to individuals with diverse life styles.

This objective suggests that this awareness is developed only in group discussions. Also, evaluation of the behavior must validate that learning occurred in group discussion. This approach is most unrealistic, for it is well known that individuals have many sources of learning and the student could have achieved this awareness through other life experiences.

A good guideline to remember when writing behavioral objectives is: when you find yourself ready to use words such as *through* or *by,* stop—because you are involving yourself with methodology.

Statements Rather Than a List of Topics

Occasionally one sees a list of topics representing theories, concepts, laws, or generalizations identified as the list of objectives for a particular educational experience. Previous discussions about behavioral objectives should indicate why such a list could not meet criteria for objectives. Objectives refer to actions expected of the learner. The topics, which in reality are content, suggest no action on the part of the learner. They offer no direction for program planning and certainly are impossible to evaluate.

What would the following list for a unit of a course mean?

Self-care

Stress and coping

Health, illness

This list tells the reader only that these topics are included in the unit. There is no clue as to the depth to which they are to be explored or to the focus of the exploration. Certainly, one has no idea what the learner is expected to do about these topics and, therefore, they cannot be evaluated. Thus, a list of topics shows the content area; it is not an objective.

Objectives as Statement of a Plan of a Course

Objectives have one major purpose—the statement of intended outcomes of an educational experience. When developed for a course or unit of instruction, they are not meant to represent the outline of that course. Indeed, strong, meaningful objectives may be addressed in many areas of a course. Often a particular learning experience may be contributing to the development of several objectives at any one time. When objectives are written for each of the three domains of learning, it is often that one experience may incorporate all three domains. As an example, teaching of injection skill will involve the cognitive objective of using principles, the psychomotor objective of performance, and the affective objective of value of the recipient of the therapy. Objectives may be listed in a sequence that has inherent logic, but the sequence should not represent the plan of the course of unit of instruction.

ANALYSIS OF A BEHAVIORAL OBJECTIVE

Behavioral objectives are to be used by educators and students. Too often the development of behavioral objectives becomes an end in itself. After one faculty group had worked for some time in developing objectives for a course and reached a consensus on the objectives, one faculty member said, "Now that we have the objectives done, let's put them away and get down to identifying the content." How often this same behavior occurs! It would seem that some faculty may know how to write behaviors but they do not know what to do with them once they are developed.

Behavioral objectives tell much. The Behavioral Objective Analysis Direction Model (Fig. 3-1) provides an approach for using general behavioral objectives as a guide in all parts of the educational endeavor. This model states that behavioral objectives give direction to:

1. The behavior called for.

2. The content designated.

Behavioral objectives provide clues to:

1. The method best suited to meet the objective. (Method is designated as the teaching activity of the teacher.)

2. The type of learning experience which enables the learner to accomplish the behavior desired in the objective. (Learning activity is designated as the activity in which the learner is involved.)

3. Methods and criteria for evaluation of the attainment of the objective.

It is in these three areas of method, learning experience, and evaluation that the opportunity for creativity and individualization of learning experience occurs. The nature of the behavior and the content suggest possible approaches in these areas. We might use as an example a behavior that is a psychomotor skill. In this case, methodology and learning experience must include a practice component, and evaluation must be through observation. However, these are not the only possible ways to follow through on this behavior, and an assortment of approaches developed in response to the clues provided by the behavior and content serve to provide variety in teaching, learning, and evaluation.

Earlier in this chapter, a general behavioral objective was presented. The analysis of that objective according to the Behavioral Objective Analysis Direction Model (Fig. 3-1) follows.

OBJECTIVE: The nursing student distinguishes the differences between male and female patterns of communication.

1. Behavior   Distinguish differences
2. Content   Communication process
                       • Elements: message, sender, receiver
                       • Means: verbal, nonverbal, graphic
                       Factors influencing the process

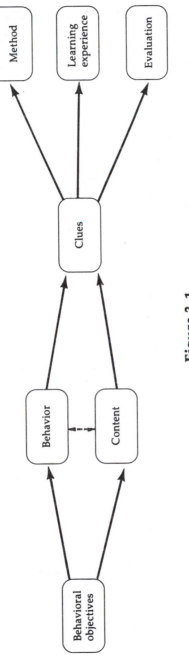

Figure 3–1
Behavioral Objective Analysis Direction Model

49

Differences in anatomical structure of male and female vocal apparatus

Influence of anatomical structure on verbal means of communication

Social and cultural influences on male and female communication patterns

CLUES

1. Method	Readings
	Questioning
	Group discussion
	Visual aids—models, transparencies, etc.
	Audiovisual aids—films, slides, tapes, recordings, videotapes
	Supervised clinical practice
	Computer-assisted instruction
	Simulations
2. Learning activity	Reading from selections on bibliography
	Listening to tapes, records
	Viewing videotapes
	Written paper
	Process recording
	Role playing
	Comparative study of male and female patient communication
	Oral presentation to peers
3. Evaluation	Clinical conference
	• Describe communication differences between male and female patients as each discussed some aspect of his or her care
	Written assignment
	• Describe differences in male and female communication as portrayed on slide tape in which a man and a woman read Rod McKuen's poem, "Knowing When to Leave"

Library reference

• Paper showing differences as noted by authorities

Process recording of a male and female patient interaction analyzed for data, interpretation, and implications.

This analysis is not intended to be comprehensive, but it does illustrate the potential for making the behavioral objective operational. Analyses of the behavioral objectives suggest content relevant for the educational experience. Identification of a variety of methods and learning activities enables faculty and students to use paths toward attaining the objective that meet the needs of particular students and learning situations. Various approaches to evaluation will increase the data base concerning a student's competency or will individualize the evaluation so that it is specific for a given learner and/or situation need.

Once identified from all behavioral objectives designated for a particular educational experience, the content can then be organized in whatever logical fashion the faculty deems appropriate. Methodology and learning experiences are then selected as indicated in the analysis. The important point is that all parts of the educational experience are related to behaviors specified as desired outcomes.

MASTERY OF LEARNING CONCEPT APPLIED TO BEHAVIORAL OBJECTIVES

One question often raised by program developers relative to behavioral objectives is: For whom should behavioral objectives be designed—the average student, the top student, or the below-average student? The answer the teacher selects has much to do with his or her attitude toward and beliefs about the teaching–learning process and expectations of the learner's performance. If the expectations predicate that a certain percentage of students will succeed, another percentage will fail, and another percentage will partially meet the objectives, the teacher's academic goals have been formalized at least in attitude and the results will be consistent with these expectations. Indeed, a self-fulfilling prophesy has been created.

Bloom (1971), in a chapter *Mastery Learning*, addresses this issue and states that given sufficient time (and appropriate types of help), "95 percent of students (the top 5 percent plus the next 90 percent) can learn a subject up to a high level of mastery" (p. 51). This conclusion is based on studies of aptitude distributions, which indicate the following three groupings of students:

1. At the top of the distribution is 1 to 5 percent with a special talent for the subject and an ability to learn it quickly and with greater fluency than other students.

2. At the other extreme is less than 5 percent with special disability for a particular learning (e.g., a person who thinks in concrete forms would have difficulty with abstract concepts in nursing).

3. In between is 90 percent where aptitudes are predictive of rate of learning rater than the level (or complexity) of learning.

The mastery of learning concept does not say that 95 percent of the students *will achieve* mastery. It says only that they have the *potential*. Five variables are relevant to this concept and may be used effectively in our formative evaluation protocols. The five variables are:

1. Aptitude for a particular type of learning, which refers to the amount of time required by the learner to attain mastery of a learning task.

2. Quality of instruction, which refers to the degree to which the presentation, explanation, and ordering of elements of the task to be learned approach optimum for a given learner.

3. Ability to understand instruction, which refers to the learner's understanding of the nature of the task to be learned and the procedure to be followed in the learning of the task.

4. Perseverance, which refers to the time the learner is willing to put into learning.

5. Time allowed for learning, which is the key to the concept of aptitude.

Should we then say that 95 percent of the learners can master a particular behavioral objective, providing a strategy for mastery of learning is developed that considers individual differences among learners and accommodates the teaching–learning process to these differences? The teacher who enters a learning situation with such a goal in mind will be ready to diagnose student needs and provide support services and teaching strategies based on the diagnosis. The teaching–learning situation then tends to become a facilitating experience for all students, rather than a satisfying one for some.

As Bloom et al. (1971) suggest, a common practice in education programs is a misuse of the statistical theory, which works against the mastery of learning approach. The normal curve, which predicates that a certain percent of students will master a learning task, an equal number will fail, and the rest will fall in a rank on a scale, is based on the notion of chance in random activity. In nursing, learners do not represent a random simple; they are a highly selective group of individuals. Since our educational endeavors for this highly selective group is purposeful activity, the results of achievement should show a skewed curve. Bloom et al. point out the fallacy in using a normal curve to depict academic competency, stating: "In fact, we may even insist that our educational efforts have been unsuccessful to the extent to which our distribution of achievement approximates the normal distribution" (p. 45).

The critical issue is not for what type of student the behavioral objectives should be developed, but rather what mastery of learning strategies should be instituted as the objectives become operational so that, except for the possible few who may have a special disability for that type of behavior, all students may succeed.

SUMMARY

Although there are several prescriptions for writing behavioral objectives, they usually can be classified into two categories, specific and general. Specific behavior objectives include:

1. Description of the learner.
2. Description of the type of behavior expected.
3. Description of the conditions under which the learner demonstrates competence.
4. A statement of an acceptable standard of performance.

General behavioral objectives include the first two components, although the second component is often stated in two elements, behavior and content.

Specific objectives are compatible with natural science theories of learning while general objectives are based on assumptions of human science theories of learning. Specific objectives are close-ended and include all the contingencies of the learning situation. As such, their use is limited primarily to learning experiences that are linear in nature and deal with part learning in an additive mode. General objectives, on the other hand, state only the behavior to be achieved and the knowledge context within which it is to occur. Since the teaching and learning strategies and evaluation methods are not included, greater flexibility to obtain the learning is gained. This freedom and opportunity challenge the participants in the learning experience to be creative and responsive to possibilities and potentials which the situation offers. The general format then is compatible with educational programs in complex fields of study where problem solving and issue confrontation require creative, clear thinking practitioners.

Since behavioral objectives serve primarily as a means of communication for all parties involved in the educational endeavor, they must be written clearly and explicitly. Behavioral terms imply action, and the actions stated must be appropriate to the situation and must be measurable.

Behavioral objectives are to be used by program planners as well as by actual participants in the teaching–learning situation. They must be analyzed in terms of behavior, content, method, learning experience, and evaluation. The results of this analysis are then synthesized into the program of instruction.

Expectations of a student's ability to meet the behavioral objective greatly influence his or her attitude and that of the teacher as they come together for the educational experience. Recognition that at least 95 percent of the learners may attain the objective challenges the teacher to diagnose learning needs and to develop mastery of learning strategies.

REFERENCES

Bloom, B. S. (Ed.). (1956). *Taxonomy of educational objectives. Handbook I: Cognitive domain.* New York: Longman.

Bloom, B. S. (1971). Mastery learning. In J. H. Block (Ed.), *Mastery learning: Theory and practice* (pp. 47–63). New York: Holt, Rinehart and Winston.

Bloom, B., Hastings, J., & Madaus, G. (1971). *Handbook on formative and summative evaluation of student learning.* New York: McGraw-Hill.

Dewey, J. (1961). *Democracy and education.* New York: Macmillan.

Durbach, E., Goodall, R., & Wilkinson, K. (1987). Instructional objectives in patient education. *Nursing Outlook, 35*(12), 82–83, 88.

Kibler, R., Barker, L., & Miles, D. (1970). *Behavioral objectives and instruction.* Boston: Allyn & Bacon.

Krathwohl, D., Bloom, B., & Masia, B. (1964). *Taxonomy of educational objectives. Handbook II: Affective domain.* New York: Longman.

Tanner, D. (1972). *Using behavioral objectives in the classroom.* New York: Macmillan.

Tyler, R. (1950). *Basic principles of curriculum and instruction.* Chicago: University of Chicago.

Whitehead, A. (1958). *The aims of education.* New York: Macmillan (Free Press).

RECOMMENDED READINGS

Bigge, M. (1982). *Learning theories for teachers* (2nd. ed.). New York: Harper & Row.

Block, J. (Ed.). (1971). *Mastery learning: Theory and practice.* New York: Holt, Rinehart & Winston.

Kliebard, H. (1975). Persistent curriculum issues in historical perspective. In W. Pinar (ED.), *Curriculum theorizing: The reconceptualists* (pp. 39–50). Berkeley: McCutchan.

Mager, R. (1962). *Preparing educational objectives.* Palo Alto: Fearon.

Reilly, D. (1981). Why objectives? Relationship to occupational nursing practice. *Occupational Health Nursing, 29*(1), 7–11.

4

Use of Taxonomy in
Developing Behavioral
Objectives for Nursing

A behavioral objective is not an isolate. It is part of a total phenomenon; as such it is related to all other behavioral objectives salient to that phenomenon. The boundaries of the phenomenon are circumscribed by some predetermined overall framework. In program planning this means that some system of ordering behavioral objectives must be utilized to provide for their interrelationship and for their expression in terms of developmental progress goals.

The system selected must answer nursing's concern for identification of levels of behavior that signify development within an educational program or relevancy to the needs of a particular group of learners. It must help program developers to identify specific behaviors that can be measured. Too often one finds such terms as *basic* knowledge, *increased* knowledge, and *greater* knowledge in statements of objectives. These adjectives, however, cannot be measured since they are not on a continuum within some acceptable framework. What is basic? Increased from what? Greater than what?

HOLISTIC NATURE OF A PERSON'S BEHAVIOR

Any system or approach to ordering behaviors according to a particular classification falls short in its ability to describe the totality of a person's behavioral responses. A person is a thinking, feeling, acting, social being who responds as a total organism to stimuli from the environment. In some instances the components of a person's behavior respond in harmony; at other times there is disunity among the components, with one or more predominating at any one time. Unity of response is wisdom, a goal toward which all learners should be directed. However, as the complexity of life interfaces with the complexity of human behavior, a person finds that the search for wisdom is a life-long process.

Failure to recognize the imbalance between components of a person's behavioral response leads to unrealistic expectations and inappropriate actions. In the health field how often have we predicated our actions on the assumption that one's rational nature predominates, and thus ignored the role of custom, habit, motivation, and perception in determining how an individual will respond to our therapeutic regimens or health teaching.

Because the individual's behavioral responses to stimuli are holistic, program planners must recognize that the behavioral objectives of programs or any unit of teaching really represent multiple behaviors. This issue will be discussed in more detail later, but as the teacher develops programs and prepares for their evaluation, there must be an acknowledgment of the multidimensional character of one's behavior.

A TAXONOMY APPROACH

A system for ordering behaviors within the context of development—one which is being stressed by educators—is the taxonomy of educational objectives developed by Bloom, Krathwohl, and their associates. The reader is referred to two publications: Bloom (1956): *Taxonomy of Educational Objectives, Handbook I: Cognitive Domain*, and Krathwohl et al. (1964): *Taxonomy of Educational Objectives, Handbook II: Affective Domain*. These sources provide specific information relative to the theoretical basis for taxonomies, the process by which they were developed, and their application in educational programs. Some general areas for discussion should be mentioned as a basis for using the taxonomies in nursing educational endeavors.

Concept of Taxonomy

A taxonomy is a classification system. Bloom (1956) developed such a system for educational goals; he conceived the taxonomy as an educational-logical-psychological classification system.

Educational: boundaries between categories to be closely related to distinctions teachers make in planning curricula and choosing learning experiences.

Logical: terms to be defined as precisely as possible and used consistently.

Psychological: concepts to be consistent with relevant and accepted psychological principles and theories (p. 6).

Taxonomy then specifies the desired outcomes of an instructional endeavor. Krathwohl et al. (1964) observe that the meaning of educational objectives could be enhanced by using a taxonomy in which an objective is placed within a large overall scheme or matrix. They state, "Here it is hoped that placing the objective within the classification scheme would locate it on a continuum and thus serve to indicate what is intended as well as what is NOT intended" (p. 4).

Rationale for Taxonomic System

The critical dimension of a taxonomic system, like the behavioral objectives themselves, is its potential for facilitating communication in matters of education to all concerned. There is a need for standardized terminology that is applicable to human behavioral responses which educators seek to evaluate. Abstract terms to describe these responses negate the possibility of evaluation.

Krathwohl et al. (1964) identify four values of a taxonomy to which he and his associates subscribed

1. *The actual sharing in the process of classifying educational objectives would help members of the group clarify and tighten the language of educational objectives.*

2. *The classification scheme would provide a convenient system for describing and ordering test items, examination techniques, and evaluation instruments.*

3. *The scheme provides a means of studying and comparing educational programs.*

4. *Principles of classifying educational outcomes could reveal a real order among outcomes* (p. 4).

Hayter (1983) cites purposes which can be accomplished by using a taxonomy system:

Increase the likelihood that educators will clarify their goals, build successively, and focus on outcomes instead of content

Help educators write objectives in the domain and level appropriate to their unique educational endeavors

Provide guidance for the selection of learning experiences appropriate for each objective and for evaluating outcomes of learning

Increase the likelihood that high level objectives will be written and accomplished (p. 340).

A taxonomy has a direct bearing on nursing programs as it helps nurse teachers assure ample high-quality objectives. Perusal of many examinations or other evaluative procedures supports the contention that recall of information is emphasized in education. Nurses *use* information, and it is their ability to use information in a variety of problem situations that should be evaluated. Likewise, in the affective domain, little if any attention is directed toward evaluating the valuing process and the internalization of values. As members of a helping profession nurses cannot remain in a state of awareness, the lowest levels of affective behavior, relative to the worth and dignity of each human being. They must value each human being and internalize their values so that their behavior lends credence to their stated values. This means that higher affective behaviors must be emphasized in the nursing program.

A faculty or group using a taxonomy, then, must select methodology, learning experiences, and evaluation procedures related to the level of behavior deemed relevant to a particular group of learners. This level is selected from the range on the continuum of the taxonomy. Tanner (1972) sees the taxonomy system as "designed to classify the intended behaviors of students as a result of participating in some set of instructional experiences, and to be used in obtaining evidence on the extent to which such behaviors are manifest" (p. 2).

Domains of Instructional Objectives

Learning behavior is manifested in three ways: (a) cognitive, the intellectual ability; (b) affective, the states of feeling, valuing; and (c) psychomotor, the manipulative and motor skills.

As described earlier in this chapter, most behavior that arises from learning is a composite of all three manifestations; yet educators have found it useful to classify instructional objectives into the three domains: cognitive, affective, and psychomotor. Kibler, Barker, and Miles (1970) suggest three reasons for this method of classifying objectives:

1. *To avoid concentrating on one or two categories to the exclusion of others.*

2. *To make sure that instruction is provided for prerequisite objectives before attempting to teach more complex ones.*

3. *To assure that appropriate instruments are employed to evaluate desired objectives* (p. 44).

Bloom (1956) and Krathwohl et al. (1964) noted the interdependence of these three domains of behavior as they developed the taxonomies, but they supported their decision for a separate taxonomy for the cognitive and the affective domains with the fact that teachers and curriculum workers do differentiate between problem solving and attitudes as well as among acting, thinking, and feeling. Recognizing that any classification scheme that attempts to order phenomena does some injustice to them, as observed in practice, Krathwohl et al. (1964) feel that the "value of these attempts to abstract and classify is in their greater powers for organizing and controlling the phenomena. We believe the value of the present system of classification is likely to be in the greater precision with which objectives are likely to be stated, in the increased communicability of the objectives, and in the extent to which evaluation evidence will become available to appropriate student progress toward the objectives" (p. 8).

Each of these domains represents a broad classification of human behavior and each is amenable to classification within its parameters on a progressive developmental continuum. Each category of behavior builds upon the skills identified in the category below it.

The identification of a specific behavioral objective within one of the behavioral domains is a professional judgment of program planners and is generally based on the decision to measure a particular skill. One has to realize, however, that these judgments do reflect the values of the planners, and care must be taken to assure that the domain selected is the proper one for a particular learning experience. Arbitrary decisions as to the classification of behavioral objectives could lead not only to emphasis on unimportant aspects of the situation, but also to emphases that are not consistent with the developmental needs of the learner.

We are what we learn. If analysis of a health problem involves only cognition of the biophysical component and ignores the nursing student's search for values as they relate to the solution of a problem, then much harm has been done to the learner. The input of self relative to feelings, beliefs, values, and attitudes must also be explored in problem-solving situations. Tanner (1972) stresses that developers of taxonomies of instructional objectives must recognize the continuity and interdependence of the three domains as he reminds the reader, ". . . it should be stressed that although the term domain implies a separation of spheres of activity, in effective learning these spheres are marked, not by separation and isolation, but by continuity and interdependence" (pp. 4, 5). He further suggests that it would be useful for teachers and curriculum workers to examine these domains separately with a view toward:

1. *Developing teaching–learning strategies and evaluative measures that are more fully representative of the broad spectrum of cognitive goals that are attainable.*

2. *Developing teaching–learning strategies that are representative of affective goals relevant to the curriculum.*

3. *Developing needed interrelationships between cognitive and affective goals in the teaching–learning process and in the evaluation of achievement* (p. 8).

Within a nursing program Tanner's list should be expanded to include:

4. *Developing teaching–learning strategies that are representative of the psychomotor competencies relevant to the practice of nursing.*

COGNITIVE DOMAIN

The cognitive domain deals with knowledge acquisition, at different levels of complexity, and the development of intellectual skills. Knowledge reflects the substantive content of nursing, inclusive of both nursing knowledge and concepts and theories derived from other disciplines, and the underlying intellectual skills inherent in nursing practice. These intellectual or cognitive skills include the processes of critical thinking, problem solving, decision making, and clinical judgment; competencies inherent in the role of health care professionals as they address the needs of their clients and profession within a complex ever changing society. They are the essential ingredients in any professional program and need to be so identified as outcome statements. The education of students in nursing requires acquisition of these intellectual skills to enable them to problem solve effectively in the clinical field, carry out the process of clinical judgment, and use nursing and related knowledge in the care of clients and delivery of that care.

Although this chapter will not review in depth the different theoretical perspectives of the cognitive processes inherent in nursing, a brief summary is included for the reader. Learning within the cognitive domain includes an understanding of concepts, principles, and theories and development of higher level intellectual skills of critical thinking, problem solving, decision making, and clinical judgment. The creative use of facts and specific information relevant to nursing practice represents an important outcome of a nursing education program. The fragile nature of facts in an information society limits their certainty, and thus student learning should emphasize concepts, principles, and theories pertinent to nursing. Concepts provide the means through which facts and specific information may be grouped together into categories. Students in the health fields are faced with a multitude of facts and details to be learned. Through concept learning, the student groups together facts and is able to categorize new information (Reilly & Oermann, 1985). In this way concepts assist learners in categorizing events or objects with which they deal in the clinical field and in the professional milieu and enable learners to organize their perceptions and experiences.

The ability to think critically is essential to the practice of nursing and functioning effectively within our complex and ever changing society. Critical thinking is rational thinking. Yinger (1980) views it as the cognitive activity associated with the evaluation of ideas. Halpern (1984) describes critical thinking as purposeful and goal directed, thereby enabling the person to solve problems and make decisions. The development of critical thinking skills has always been important but is particularly acute today when the "output of information far exceeds our ability to think critically about that information" (Meyers, 1986, p. xi). The information explosion in the health field and complexity of client problems demand ability to think critically in order to recognize the problems to be solved and decide upon actions to be taken.

Critical thinking represents the thought process that underlies problem solving, decision making, and clinical judgment; these intellectual processes all require rational thinking. In a discussion of critical thinking in the nursing curriculum, Miller and Malcolm (1990) suggest that the ability to think critically is "an inherent cognitive activity in the process of forming clinical judgments" (p. 69). Its development among nursing students requires teaching strategies which promote inquiry and questioning, examination of different approaches, and evaluation of own ideas and those of others. Teaching methods should provide an opportunity for the learner to engage in independent thought, and should emphasize the thought processes used by students as they problem solve, make decisions, and arrive at clinical judgments. Meyers (1986) suggests that critical thinking is discipline specific; it varies from discipline to discipline. Nurses, for instance, may engage in critical thinking differently than sociologists or philosophers. While critical thinking may differ across disciplines, educators in all fields have responsibility for assisting learners in developing this skill using whatever strategies are appropriate considering the discipline.

Critical thinking cannot be developed through one individual assignment or as an outcome of one nursing course. Just as nursing students will not become proficient in taking vital signs through practice in the learning laboratory only or skilled in documentation merely by related experiences in one nursing course, so too must they be taught and practice critical thinking throughout the nursing program. Students must be challenged to think critically in all their nursing courses and clinical experiences.

Meyers (1986) believes that the teacher must present a framework for critical thinking, "a structure for making sense of the materials, issues, and methodologies" (p. 6) of the field being taught, as well as assist students in developing an attitude toward the subject which encourages analytical thought. The latter element in critical thinking reflects the inclination of the learner to ask questions, examine problems, consider different perspectives, and identify and struggle with issues. In development of this attitudinal element, the teacher must encourage and support the learner in expressing ideas and questioning long-standing approaches to problems.

In caring for clients, practitioners are continually confronted with problems to be solved including those related to clients as well as setting-oriented dilemmas requiring resolution. Some problems are relatively easy to solve while others are more complex and require a greater knowledge base for application in identifying the problem setting, problem, or solutions. Problem solving begins with an identification of the problem and proceeds through collecting and interpreting information about the problem, examining possible solutions and implications of each, and testing the solutions chosen. Problem solving is influenced by the learner's knowledge base and past experiences with similar problems. The need for skill in problem solving increases as nurses assume a greater role in health care in society and the delivery of that care and continue to practice in expanded and varied roles.

Another cognitive skill inherent in nursing practice is decision making. Nurses continually make decisions about clients, staff, the setting, and other dimensions of practice. Decisions are made throughout the problem-solving process. Decisions reflect making a choice among different alternatives after examining each, considering consequences of each, and weighing them to arrive at a judgment as to which one is most effective.

In caring for clients, the nurse continually makes decisions as to nursing diagnoses and interventions. Clinical judgment is viewed typically as a series of decisions made by the nurse: (a) decisions as to what data to collect, (b) interential decisions for interpreting the data and determining nursing diagnoses, and (c) decisions as to nursing management (Tanner, 1983). In nursing practice these decisions are inherent in the nursing process. Early views of the nursing process described it as a linear, step-by-step process; current thinking, however, acknowledges that the stages of the nursing process are interrelated and involve more complex thinking processes than originally believed. Expertise in clinical judgment is essential to effective nursing and, as such, represents a critical skill to be developed within a nursing program. Research in this area, however, is limited, although there is a growing body of literature dealing with clinical judgments and how they are arrived at by nurses. In a review of the literature, Tanner (1987) identified only 19 research studies from 1966 to 1986.

In general, theory and research suggest that the nurse initially attends to patient and other cues in the environment, generates tentative diagnostic hypotheses as possible explanations for them, collects data about the hypotheses to rule them in or out, and evaluates each hypothesis to decide on the nursing diagnoses (Oermann, 1991). Other decisions pertain to nursing management.

The process of clinical judgment has been viewed within different theoretical perspectives: (a) information processing theory, (b) decision theory, and (c) phenomenology. Regardless of the theoretical approach, clinical judgment is recognized as a complex process through which the nurse arrives at decisions as to nursing diagnoses and appropriate actions (Reilly & Oermann, 1985). Further research is needed to understand more completely this complex thinking process and relevant teaching strategies for assisting students in developing this skill.

In teaching in the cognitive domain, the faculty is concerned with assisting students in the use of knowledge, in a creative purposeful manner, and the progressive development of cognitive skills. The taxonomy of the cognitive domain represents a system for ordering cognitive behaviors from simple recall of facts and specific information to higher level cognitive skills involved in analysis, synthesis, and evaluation. The taxonomy is organized according to this principle of increasing complexity and accommodates the developmental process in acquiring skills of critical thinking, problem-solving, decision making, and clinical judgment.

Bloom (1956) describes six levels in cognitive taxonomy each with specific sublevels except for one, application. A condensed version of the *Taxonomy of Educational Objectives. Handbook I: Cognitive Domain* developed by Bloom follows. Included is a brief description of the meaning of the levels and an illustration of a behavioral objective for each one. The term *nursing student* used in the behavioral objective refers to any learner in nursing, whether engaged in a formal educational, staff development, or continuing education program. It is suggested that before the taxonomy is used as a conceptual framework for developing cognitive objectives, the original source be reviewed so as to maintain the integrity of the taxonomy as it is translated into an educational program.

The cognitive taxonomy provides a framework for selecting the appropriate level of learning in the cognitive domain and writing open-ended objectives at that level. In using the taxonomy, the teacher decides first on the desired level to be attained, then develops objectives to reflect learning at that particular level. The decision as to which level in the taxonomy to specify as the outcome of the experience is based on the teacher's own judgment considering the background and level of the learner, behavior to be achieved and its complexity, and experiences and time available for achieving that objective (Reilly & Oermann, 1985).

CONDENSED VERSION OF TAXONOMY OF COGNITIVE DOMAIN OF EDUCATIONAL OBJECTIVES*

Knowledge (Information)

1.00 *Knowledge*
Recall of specifics, universals, the recall of methods, processes, or the recall of a pattern, structure, or setting.

  1.10 *Knowledge of Specific*
Recall of specific and isolated bits of information, with emphasis on symbols with concrete referents.

    1.11 *Knowledge of Terminology*
Knowledge of the referents for specific symbols (verbal and nonverbal).

      Objective
The nursing student defines the term *adaptation*.

---

* This condensed version is presented with permission of publisher, David McKay, from Bloom, B.S. (ed.), Engelhart, M.D., Furst, E.J., Hill, W.H., and Krathwohl, D.R. *Taxonomy of Educational Objectives*: Handbook I, Cognitive Domain. New York: David McKay, 1956.

1.12 *Knowledge of Specific Facts*
Knowledge of dates, events, persons, places, source of information, properties, and phenomena.

Objective
The nursing student names the four chambers of the heart.

1.20 *Knowledge of Ways and Means of Dealing with Specifics*
Recall of ways of organizing, studying, judging, and criticizing—chiefly in passive awareness of material rather than ability to use it.

1.21 *Knowledge of Conventions*
Knowledge of characteristic ways of treating and presenting ideas and phenomena.

Objective
The nursing student identifies three ways by which nurses provide for the safety of the patient in a hospital setting.

1.22 *Knowledge of Trends and Sequences*
Knowledge of the processes, directions, and movements of phenomena with respect to time.

Objective
The nursing student identifies four trends in society that may influence the direction of the nursing profession in the future.

1.23 *Knowledge of Classifications and Categories*
Knowledge of the classes, sets, divisions, and arrangements regarded as fundamental for a given subject field, purpose, argument, or problem.

Objective
The nursing student names the classification of needs according to Maslow's hierarchy of human needs.

1.24 *Knowledge of Criteria*
Knowledge of the criteria by which facts, principles, opinions, and conducts are tested or judged.

Objective
The nursing student lists criteria to be used in assessing the effectiveness of an interview with a patient.

1.25 *Knowledge of Methodology*
Knowledge of methods of inquiry, techniques, and procedures employed in a particular subject field as well as those employed in investigating particular problems and phenomena.

Objective
The nursing student lists methods of data collection appropriate to assessing health needs of an individual.

1.30   *Knowledge of the Universals and Abstractions in a Field*
Recall of knowledge of the major ideas, schemes, and patterns by which phenomena and ideas are organized, such as theories and generalizations used in explaining phenomena and in solving problems.

   1.31   *Knowledge of Principles and Generalizations*
   Knowledge of particular abstractions that summarize observations of phenomena, i.e., explain, predict, describe, or determine most appropriate action.

   Objective
   The nursing student lists the scientific principles relevant to proper use of the sphygmomanometer in reading blood pressure.

   1.32   *Knowledge of Theories and Structures*
   Knowledge of the body principles and generalizations, together with their interrelations, present a clear, rounded, and systematic view of a complex phenomenon, problem, or field.

   Objective
   The nursing student lists two theories of stress that may be used to interpret one's behavior in a stressful situation.

Comprehension

2.00   *Comprehension*
The first level of intellectual skills relevant to understanding. At this level the learner grasps the meaning of the communicated message sufficiently well to use it in relating to other material or in solving a problem without necessarily recognizing its fullest implication.

2.10   *Translation*
The expression of the communication in another language, into other terms, or into another form of communication.

   Objective
   The nursing student gives an illustration of a nonverbal behavior that impedes effective communication between the nurse and the client.

2.20 *Interpretation*
The explanation or summary of a communication involving a rearrangement or a new perspective of the material.

Objective
The nursing student explains the aging process according to Erikson's theory of growth and development.

2.30 *Extrapolation*
The extension of trends or tendencies beyond given data and findings of the document to determine implications, consequences, corollaries, effects, etc., which are in accordance with conditions as literally described in the original communication.

Objective
The nursing student predicts the effects of a therapeutic nursing intervention for a selected health problem from data collected about patients' health needs.

Application

3.00 *Application*
The intellectual skill referring to *use* of knowledge. It is the use of abstractions, such as ideas, principles, or theories in concrete situations.

Objective
The nursing student uses the nursing process in the care of individuals and groups within the health care setting.

Analysis

4.00 *Analysis*
Emphasis on the breakdown of material into its own constituent parts and detection of the relationship of parts and of the way they are organized. Deals with content and form of material, i.e., analysis of *meaning*. Uses resources outside of data at hand.

4.10 *Analysis of Elements*
Identification of elements of a communication, the overt and covert elements, differentiating nature of the statements such as facts, value, intent.

Objective

The nursing student identifies the measures used in meeting the survival needs of the patient in cardiac crisis.

4.20   *Analysis of Relationships*

The connections and interactions between elements and parts of a communication to include relationships between different kinds of evidence, consisting of part to part, element to element, relevance of elements or parts to central idea or thesis in the communication.

Objective

The nursing student contrasts the adaptive needs of the patient in a temporary acute illness with those of a patient with a progressive illness.

4.30   *Analysis of Organization Principles*

The organization, systematic arrangement and structure which hold a communication together.

Objective

The nursing student analyzes the organizational structure of a nursing department in terms of its implications for practice.

Synthesis

5.00   *Synthesis*

The putting together of elements and parts so as to form a whole, a pattern or structure not clearly there before.

5.10   *Production of a Unique Communication*

The development of a communication reflecting the student's perspective about some ideas, attitudes, etc.

Objective

The nursing student writes an essay depicting a position relative to the expanded care responsibilities of the nurse.

5.20   *Production of a Plan or Proposed Set of Operations*

The development of a plan of work or proposal of a plan of operations.

Objective

The nursing student proposes a plan for optimizing the use of the pediatric nurse clinician in a community setting.

5.30 *Derivation of a Set of Abstract Relations*
The development of a scheme for classifying or explaining certain data or phenomena or the deduction of propositions and relations from a set of basic propositions or symbolic representations.

Objective
The nursing student formulates a theoretical framework of nursing applicable to the health care of a family that resides in an inner city environment.

Evaluation

6.00 *Evaluation*
Judgments about value for the purpose of ideas, works, solutions, methods, materials, etc. Qualitative and quantitative judgments about extent to which material and methods satisfy criteria, which are either determined by the student or given to him.

6.10 *Judgments in Terms of Internal Evidence*
The evaluation of a communication or situation from such evidence as logical accuracy, consistency, and other internal criteria.

Objective
The nursing student validates own research study in terms of internal criteria which include clarity, accuracy, validity, rehability, precision of statements, and logic of conclusions from data and appropriate documentation.

6.20 *Judgments in Terms of External Criteria*
The evaluation of a communication or situation with reference to selected criteria as comparing a work against the highest known standards in its field

Objective
The nursing student validates own research study in relation to valid and reliable studies in related areas.

The taxonomy provides a continuum reflecting a progressive development of cognitive skills that can be useful to nurse educators. The emphasis on higher level intellectual skills should characterize the outcome of programs for professional students and practitioners. For programs preparing nurses at a technical level of practice, objectives are written for a lower level of the taxonomy, at least to the application level.

AFFECTIVE DOMAIN

Few individuals will challenge the concept of behavioral objective development for the cognitive or psychomotor domains of learning, but instructors are less responsive to the notion of preparing behavioral objectives for the affective domain. Affective competencies relate to the use of moral reasoning in decisions for the management of moral and ethical dilemmas and to the development of a value system that guides decisions and activities within the individual's and society's notion of what is right and good (Reilly & Oermann, 1985). These are the competencies that characterize nursing as a humanistic and caring practice.

Contemporary society with its ambiguities, conflicting currents, and rapid change challenges the moral and ethical fiber of nursing. A most significant trend in contemporary American society which affects teaching in the affective domain is the changing character of its people as American society becomes increasingly pluralistic with the influx of new immigrants. Henry (1990), in his article, "Beyond the Melting Pot," in *Time* magazine projects that with present trends in the 21st century racial and ethnic groups in the United States will outnumber whites for the first time. With the increase in multivariate cultural groups in the society, a pluralism of value systems will occur as each group seeks to maintain its own values while bringing them into accord with the larger society. Each group has its own meaning for such concepts as health, illness, sick role, family, and so forth. Reilly (1989) reminds persons in the health fields that they must respect this diversity in meanings and practices among the groups as they provide care to each individual.

In the educational preparation of nurses, therefore, there is a demand that the program prepare practitioners capable of meeting such challenges with integrity and commitment to professional values. The old model of teaching values by fiat or precept is no longer relevant to decision making in today's more complex value situations.

There are two critical dimensions in teaching the affective domain: cognition which emphasizes skills in making choices and consistency in patterns of behavior in accord with the selected choice. Affective competency development is an integral part of the educational schema for nursing and, as such, its development is subject to the same pedagogy as the other two domains of learning, cognitive and psychomotor. This means that any program of studies for nursing includes a deliberate protocol for teaching affective competencies: statement of objectives, teaching strategies, learning experiences and evaluation methods, both formative and summative.

There are several concepts included in the rubric of affective domain that must be understood by those persons involved in teaching this domain.

Beliefs are perceptions of reality that have significance and meaning to an individual whether or not they are substantiated by fact. They impact on behavior but are often not reliable; they are vulnerable to forces operating in a situation at any point in time.

Values are judgments of worth or preference which are held by an individual. Davis and Aroskar's (1984) description is: "values may be considered to be a set of beliefs or attitudes for which logical reasons can be given. Values are significant because they influence perception, guide in actions and have consequences" (p. 197). Values are always contextual within a group or society standard. Moral values are those in accord with ethical and moral standards which refer to the good of the greater society with protection of individual rights within society (Reilly & Oermann, 1985).

Raths et al. (1966) accept the concept of values as incorporating two dimensions, choice and consistent behavior pattern. Their theory proposes three essential processes for a perception to be considered to be a value.

Choosing	(1) *freely*
	(2) *from alternatives*
	(3) *after thoughtful consideration of the consequences of each alternative*
Prizing	(4) *cherishing, happy with choice*
	(5) *willing to affirm the choice publically*
Action	(6) *doing something with the choice*
	(7) *repeatedly in some pattern of life* (pp. 28–30).

A value, as stated in this theory, requires that all criteria be met. Thus, concepts like feeling, attitude, belief, and aspirations are not values, for all three criteria are not satisfied. They are value indicators, however, and can be used by the teacher to help the student associate them with values.

Attitudes are feelings for or against a person, object, or event whose rationale may or may not be understood by the person. They do not meet all of the criteria of a value, and thus are vulnerable to changes in internal or external forces in the environment.

Moral Reasoning is the cognitive process of analysis and interpretation of a moral dilemma as a means for determining some course of action. Moral reasoning is dependent on critical thinking skill when a situation is evident for which usual rules of conduct are not sufficient. There is no assurance, however, that the decision revealed will be followed through into action. Kohlberg's (1981) work is most familiar in this field.

Ethics refers to standards of conduct of right behavior based on moral judgment. Churchill (1982) views ethics as a systematic reflection of moral behavior; morality as the practical activity, ethics as the theoretical reflective activity. Stent (1977) endorses the notion that ethics "is a human intellectual discipline which develops the principles which account for morality and moral action and the normative principles and values that guide human action" (p. 243).

Morality is perceived within a social context and is a system of moral conduct adopted by a society, community, cultural group, profession, etc. The ethical standards and values to be respected by members are declared and sanctions are instituted when deviation occurs.

The fundamental competency in the affective domain is the skill in making choices; making decisions from alternatives as to the course of action. The ability to make decisions is basic to our humanness. Dubos (1981) affirms this position, "We are human beings, not so much because of our appearance, but because of what we do, the way we do it and more importantly, because of what we elect to do or not do" (p. 9). This point is elaborated when he says, "Intentionality and freedom of choice are at least as important in human life as is biological determination" (p. 15). Frankl (1963), affirms that individuals do have freedom to choose a course of action. "There is sufficient proof that everything can be taken from a man but one thing—the last of the human freedoms—to choose one's attitude in any given set of circumstances to choose one's way" (p. 105).

Choice making in the affective domain is more than stating a preference. It is the ability to ponder evidence, examine assumptions, make judgments, and evaluate. It results in the statement of a position; it declares what a person will stand up for. Podeschi (1976) states the following about James' position on making choices. "The individual who believes that choices really matter will take life seriously. What we freely choose to do makes a difference; real issues are at stake. This means the willingness to live with energy, though energy brings pain" (p. 228).

Teaching in the affective domain requires that the objective of choice making be stated and that appropriate learning experiences be provided. Choice making is more than problem solving, however. It has an emotional component of commitment that is essential; for the decision must be translated into a constant pattern of behavior. Evaluation then addresses both the choice-making skill and the consistency in the subsequent pattern of behavior.

What values are taught? Some faculty do not desire to teach this domain for there is fear that such teaching is indoctrination and that it is inappropriate to impose one's values on another. Since values are learned, and no learning can be imposed from the outside because only the learner can learn, there is no need for concern about forcing a teacher's values on a student. The legitimate values that are appropriately a part of the education for nursing are found in the professional documents discussed below.

The *Bill of Rights of the United States Constitution* states those dimensions of a person's life which must be respected by society if justice is to prevail. Cranston (1983) reminds us that human rights are something everyone has, they are not earned, they belong to the individual because that person is a human being.

The *Code for Nurses*, first developed in 1950 and subsequently revised with the 1976 edition, provides a guide for the resolution of ethical dilemmas. An underlying theme of the dignity and worth of each human being prevails. The Code also addresses the accountability of the nurse to the profession. Toulmin (1977) reminds professionals of the inherent limitation of professional codes because individuals often have many roles, some of which may be at variance with others. Thus, codes of professional responsibilities are framed to minimize risks of recurrent obligations, but each conflict must be examined carefully.

The *Standards of Practice* (American Nurses' Association, 1973) are proposed by the professional organization and reflect the belief in the rights of clients to maintain their dignity in all encounters with the health care system.

The *Social Policy Statement of the American Nurses' Association* (1980) addresses the social context of nursing and the scope of its practice, with emphasis on the commitment and responsibilities of nurses to those whom they serve as clients or to society itself.

All three professional documents have a common theme: commitment to the dignity and worth of each person and accountability to society for quality performance. These concepts are now receiving emphasis by our nurse researchers, such as Watson (1985) and Benner and Wrubel (1989) in their research and development of a nursing model based on the phenomenon of care.

If the affective domain is perceived to be a legitimate and indispensable domain of learning, then behavioral objectives must be identified and so stated. These objectives must lend themselves to analysis in terms of behavior, content, method of teaching learning experiences, and evaluation.

Krathwohl et al. (1964) accepted the legitimacy of behavioral objectives in the affective realm and adopted the concept that affective behaviors could be developed when appropriate learning experiences were provided. Their search for an organizing principle that would enable continuum of development led to the principle of internalization: "a process by which a given phenomenon or value passed from a level of bare awareness to a position of some power to guide or control the behavior of the person" (p. 27). This process really refers to that inner growth of the individual by which is developed a value system which guides behavior in making choices for action. The hierarchy proposed by Krathwohl et al. reflects the seven criteria proposed by Raths et al. (1966) for both require that intellect and emotion blend.

Raths et al. (1966) provide the value development theory; the Code for Nurses, Standards of Practice, and Social Policy Statement identify the values inherent in nursing practice; and Krathwohl et al. (1964) provide the affective domain taxonomy which enable the program planner to state affective behaviors according to a sequencing which leads to internalization. The first two levels of the taxonomy relate to value indicators. It is at the third level, valuing, that the choice is made and internalization begins.

Following is a condensed version of the *Taxonomy of the Affective Domain* as developed by Krathwohl et al. (1964). It includes a brief description of the meaning of terms and an illustration of a behavioral objective for each level.

CONDENSED VERSION OF TAXONOMY OF AFFECTIVE DOMAIN OF EDUCATIONAL OBJECTIVES*

Receiving

1.0 *Receiving (Attending)*
Sensitivity to the existence of a given condition, phenomenon, situation, or problem.

1.1 *Awareness*
Conscious recognition of the existence of a given condition, phenomenon, situation, or problem. Individual's attention is attracted to stimuli but there is no requirement to evaluate or verbalize.

Objective
The nursing student expresses an awareness of the need to involve the patient and family in developing a plan of care.

1.2 *Willingness to Receive*
A willingness to give attention to or note a phenomenon rather than to avoid it. Response is neutral and judgment is suspended.

Objective
The nursing student listens willingly to the patient express concerns.

---

* The condensed version is presented with permission of publisher, David McKay, from Krathwohl, D.R., Bloom, B.S., Masia, B.B. *Taxonomy of Educational Objectives*, Handbook II: Affective Domain. New York David McKay, 1968.

1.3   *Controlled or Selected Action*
Differentiation, selection, or discrimination among various aspects of a phenomenon. Involves differentiation of aspects of stimuli and/ or attention to certain stimuli. Favored stimulus is selected and attended to.

Objective
The nursing student notes comments made by nurses that suggest stereotypic views of various categories of people.

2.0   *Responding*
Reacting overtly to a stimulus or phenomenon, and doing something with or about them.

2.1   *Acquiescence in Responding*
Complying with expectations, especially of those individuals in authority.

Objective
The nursing student reads the required references listed in the course bibliography.

2.2   *Willingness to Respond*
Voluntary action in response to a given phenomenon reflecting a choice for the action.

Objective
The nursing student seeks opportunities for the mother of a sick child to participate in care.

2.3   *Satisfaction in Response*
Enjoyment in acting on or responding to a given phenomenon. Emotional significance is now being attached to the stimulus.

Objective
The nursing student shares readily with peers experiences in interacting with patients and families.

Valuing

3.0   *Valuing*
A step in the internalization process signified by the attachment of worth or belief. Behavior is sufficiently consistent and stable to be characteristic of a belief or attitude.

3.1 *Acceptance of a Value*
Belief in a phenomenon, behavior, object, etc., with reasonable certainty and sufficient internalization to be a controlling force. A willingness to be identified as one holding that belief.

Objective
The nursing student supports the rights of individuals to their own philosophies, moral codes, and life styles.

3.2 *Preference for a Value*
A willingness to pursue or seek out activities related to a phenomenon or belief that one has attached worth to and therefore is willing to be identified with.

Objective
The nursing student assumes responsibility for involving patients and their families in decisions of care that affect their lives.

3.3 *Commitment*
Belief with a high degree of certainty leading to conviction and involvement in the cause, principle, or doctrine. The individual is perceived as holding the value and motivated to act out the behavior.

Objective
The nursing student acts in an advocate role when patients' human rights are threatened in a patient care setting.

Organization

4.0 *Organization*
Development of values into an organized system after considering their interrelationships and establishing value priorities.

4.1 *Conceptualization of a Value*
The quality of abstraction or conceptualization is added to stability and consistency. Relationship between a value and the ones already held or new is involved.

Objective
The nursing student formulates judgments about nursing responsibilities relative to extraordinary means of maintaining life in a critically ill patient.

4.2 *Organization of a Value System*
Development of a complex of values, including disparate ones, into an ordered relationship that is both harmonious and internally consistent.

Relationship of values is more likely to be described as a kind of dynamic equilibrium that is, in part, dependent upon portions of the environment relevant at any point in time.

Objective
The nursing student formulates a plan of action consistent with professional values when confronted with decisions involving moral issues relevant to quality of life.

Characterization by a Value or Value Complex

5.0 *Characterization by a Value or Value Complex*
Internalization of a philosophy of life resulting from internalization of values; organization of an internally consistent system of values; and a consistent behavior pattern so that the individual is described in terms of his unique personal characteristics. The relationship between cognitive and affective processes is pronounced.

5.1 *Generalized Set*
Basic orientation that enables individual to reduce and order the complex world about him/her and to act consistently and effectively in it.

Objective
The nursing student judges health care problems in terms of issues, purposes, situations, and consequences rather than fixed dogmatic precepts, stereotypic ideas, and emotional wishful thinking.

5.2 *Characterization*
Internalization of a value system having as its object the whole of what is known, or knowable, with an internal consistency.

Objective
The nursing student develops a philosophy of life based on a personal and professional code of ethics that denotes his or her participation in improving the health and welfare of all members of society.

The taxonomy described here presents a hierarchy of value development toward the ultimate goal of self-actualization. Individuals will be at different stages of the internalization process relative to different values at any point in time. Development is not a static process in which a value becomes permanently entrenched, but rather one that subjects the value to constant analysis and testing as the individual is called upon to make behavioral decisions in a world that is constantly changing.

PSYCHOMOTOR DOMAIN

A taxonomy for the psychomotor domain of learning has not been developed to the level of sophistication and utility found in other domains, perhaps because in the literature there is less evidence of objectives written for this type of competency. Nonetheless, psychomotor skills are significant in nursing practice where they are found in both the assessment and intervention stages of the nursing process. Psychomotor skills are those domains of nursing practice that entail the ability to behave efficiently in action situations that require neuromuscular coordination (Reilly & Oermann, 1985). Singer (1975) states, "activities that are primarily movement oriented and that emphasize overt physical response bear the label, psychomotor" (p. 23).

Psychomotor skills involve all three domains of learning: cognitive which relates to knowledge of principles, relationships and processes; affective which in use of the skill conveys recognition of value and worth of the recipient of care and professional integrity of the caregiver; and psychomotor which relates to coordination of action and precision in performance. Although all three domains are integrated in the competency, each domain can be examined separately, for different teaching and evaluation strategies are entailed.

Three types of skill have been identified (Reilly & Oermann, 1985):

1. *Fine motor skills: muscular coordination involves precision-oriented tasks. Nursing skills include injection, arterial line manipulation, and surgical dressings requiring instrumentation.*

2. *Manual skills: manipulative tasks that are fairly repetitive and usually involve eye-arm action. Nursing skills include: physical assessment, body hygiene, suctioning, chest drainage, and touch.*

3. *Gross motor skills: involve large muscles and movement of the body. Nursing skills include: cardiopulmonary resuscitation, range of motion, and patient positioning.*

Singer (1975) identifies characteristics for the skilled person:

1. *Performance is fairly consistent regardless of factors present that might cause the "average" person's performance to fluctuate.*

2. *Performance coincides with high degree of spatial precision and timing.*

3. *Responses to stimuli are set in appropriate sequential order.*

4. *Performances are executed within certain time limitations.*

5. *Ability to anticipate quickly is present and there is more time to react.*

6. *Performance has less variability since there is no need to respond to every potential cue in the environment.*

7. *Ability to receive maximum information from minimum number of identifiable cues is developed* (p. 29).

There is a misconception among some educators that because psychomotor skills are observable behaviors, the theoretical basis for teaching them is derived from behaviorism. Much research in the field negates such a premise for behavioral cybernetic models, information processing models, and adaptation models have been developed to explain the complex mental and physical processes involved in psychomotor skill development. Learning in this domain is cognitive, not mechanistic, with emphasis on the physiologic, psychologic, and cognitive processes that occur within the organism in response to cues from the environment, resulting in a coordinated and effective performance.

Practice is an essential component of psychomotor skill learning with the nature and the amount dependent on multiple factors: the goal to be achieved; the degree of complexity of the skill to be mastered; individual characteristics of the learner; and situation variables which impact on the learning process (Reilly & Oermann, 1985). Research by Martenuik (1969) and Henry (1958) indicates that there is no such element as generalized motor ability, but rather motor learning ability is task specific and dependent on such other factors as innate ability, previous learning, motivation and other variables. Fleishman (1972), Kelso (1982), and Singer (1975) report research that suggests the ability of a person to respond to stimuli and select relevant cues is a function of a person's perceptual style. Burton (1976) conducted research relative to perceptual style using three patterns of practice for learning the fine complex skill of subcutaneous injection. The three patterns were: mental (visualizing task), physical, and a combination of physical and mental. Results show that field-independent learners learn the skill regardless of the pattern more readily than do field-dependent learners. As a matter of fact, the performance of field-dependent learners deteriorated when the combination pattern was used. Burton's (1976) explanation states, "In learning skills, perceptual awareness of bodily kinesthetic cues and appropriate response to these contributes to mastery of skill regardless of practice used" (p. 73). Much research has been conducted relative to practice modalities, but cannot be included here. The reader is referred to Reilly and Oermann (1985) and cited original sources to examine this research further.

Suffice to say, psychomotor skill learning is a complex process demanding far more knowledge than suggested by the simple mechanistic behavioral approach. The search for a taxonomy which would enable teachers to focus on the orderly process of neuromuscular development led to the taxonomy proposed by Dave (1970) which refers to those behaviors which include muscular action and require neuromuscular coordination. The organizing principle of the taxonomy is coordination. Simpson's (1966) taxonomy although often mentioned in the literature did not meet the need for a taxonomy comparable to those produced for the other domains, for a single unifying principle related to neuromuscular performance is not evident. The steps in Simpson's taxonomy are: perception, set, guided response, mechanism, and complex overt response.

Dave's (1970) taxonomy is presented below. It does not have the authenticity of the taxonomies of the other two domains of learning, but research should determine its reliability and validity. Five major steps are identified. With refinement, interim steps could be suggested as occurs with other taxonomies.

PSYCHOMOTOR LEVELS*

1.0   *Imitation*

When the learner is exposed to an observable action, he/she begins to make covert imitation of that action. Such covert behavior appears to be the starting point in the growth of psychomotor skill. This is then followed by overt performance of an act and capacity to repeat it.

Interpretation

This behavior would be the learner's first experience following a demonstration by the nursing instructor or a viewing of a demonstration on a film or videotape.

Objective

The nursing student uses the sphygmomanometer to obtain a blood pressure reading on a patient.

2.0   *Manipulation*

Developing skill in following directions, performing selected actions, and fixing performance through necessary practice are emphasized.

Interpretation

At this stage the learner would be familiar with a written nursing procedure and would be able to use it as a guide in carrying out a skill.

Objective

The nursing student takes the patient's blood pressure reading, according to accepted procedure.

* By Dr. R.H. Dave, Head of Department of Curriculum and Evaluation, National Institute of Education, NIE Building, Nehraul Road, New Delhi.

3.0 *Precision*
Performance efficiency of a given act reaches a higher level of refinement. The learner performs the skill independent of a model or set of directions.

Interpretation
At this stage the learner is secure enough to carry out the skill independently with a high degree of accuracy.

Objective
The nursing student takes a patient's blood pressure reading accurately and in a manner consistent with scientific principles.

4.0 *Articulation*
Coordination of a series of acts is emphasized by establishing an appropriate sequence, achieving harmony or internal consistency among different acts.

Interpretation
This is the stage at which the learner blends all of the steps and variables bearing upon a skill. The skill is carried out smoothly within a reasonable time frame. Coordination is achieved.

Objective
The nursing student measures the patient's blood pressure competently, according to criteria of accuracy, smoothness, and reasonableness of time.

5.0 *Naturalization*
A high level of proficiency is required to perform a single act skillfully. The act is performed with the least expenditure of psychic energy. It is routinized to such an extent that it becomes an automatic and spontaneous response.

Interpretation
This is the stage at which the nursing learner shifts focus relative to psychomotor skill. The skill becomes a means to an end rather than an end in itself.

Objective
The nursing student integrates the taking of a patient's blood pressure reading into total therapeutic plan for that patient.

Reilly and Oermann (1985) propose performance criteria for each level of the taxonomy that are compatible with Singer's (1975) characteristics of a skilled person.

P1.0   *Imitation*

Observed actions are followed.

Movements are gross.

Coordination lacks smoothness.

Errors are present.

Time and speed are based on learner needs.

P2.0   *Manipulation*

Written instructions are followed.

Coordination of movements is variable.

Accuracy is in terms of written prescription.

Time and speed are variable.

P3.0   *Precision*

A logical sequence of actions is carried out.

Coordination is at a high level.

Errors are minimal and do not involve critical actions.

Time and speed are variable.

P4.0   *Articulation*

A logical sequence of actions is carried out.

Coordination is at a high level.

Errors are generally limited.

Time and speed are within reasonable expectations.

P5.0   *Naturalization*

Sequence of actions is automatic.

Coordination is consistently at a high level.

Time and speed are within reality.

Performance reflects professional competence.

These criteria reflect the development of psychomotor skill competency. The taxonomy suggests that accuracy should be stressed before speed. The final stage describes performance whereby the individual is no longer concerned about the "how-to-do" of the skill, for it has become an integral part of nursing practice and is retrieved upon appropriate cues. It is at this point when the cognitive, psychomotor, and affective domains have become integrated for a competent performance.

This taxonomy, like those in the other domains, enables a faculty to specify objectives at the appropriate level for the students and the particular point in the curriculum plan. With this particular taxonomy, some psychomotor skills will reach the fifth stage within the framework of one course, while others may extend over several school terms. Indeed a curriculum plan may indicate that for some skills, only the second or third level will be achieved because of the infrequency of the use of the skill in practice, thus limiting practice potential. The selected level is a function of the professional judgment of the faculty.

Table 4–1 presents verbs appropriate for each level of the three taxonomies.

TABLE 4–1
Behavioral Verbs Appropriate for
Each Level of the Three Taxonomies

I. Cognitive

    C1.0 Knowledge (Information)

define	name
identify	recall
list	recognize

    C2.0 Comprehension

        C2.1 Translation level

cite examples of	give in own words

        C2.2 Interpretation level

choose	discriminate
demonstrate use of	explain
describe	interpret
differentiate	select

        C2.3 Extrapolation level

conclude	estimate
detect	infer
determine	predict
draw conclusions	

    C3.0 Application

apply	generalize
develop	relate
employ	use

    C4.0 Analysis

appraise	detect
compare	distinguish
contrast	evaluate
criticize	identify
deduce	problem solve
	think critically

    C5.0 Synthesis

classify	produce
create	reconstruct
design	restructure

TABLE 4-1 (continued)

C5.0   Synthesis
        develop   synthesize
        modify   systematize
        organize

  C6.0 Evaluation
        appraise   evaluate
        assess   judge
        critique   validate

II. Affective

  A1.0 Receiving
        acknowledge   show awareness of
        share

  A2.0 Responding
        act willingly   practice
        discuss willingly   respond
        express satisfaction in   seek opportunities
        is willing to support   select
        listen to   show interest

  A3.0 Valuing
        accept   cooperate with
        acclaim   help
        agree   participate in
        assist   respect
        assume responsibility   support

  A4.0 Organization of Values
        argue   formulate a position
        debate   is consistent
        declare   take a stand
        defend

  A5.0 Characterization by Value
        act consistently   stand for
        is accountable

III. Psychomotor

  P1.0 Imitation
        follow example of
        follow lead of

  P2.0 Manipulation
        carry out according   follow procedure
        to procedure   practice

  P3.0 Precision
        demonstrate skill in using

  P4.0 Articulation
        carry out   use
        is skillful in using

  P5.0 Naturalization
        is competent   carry out competently
        is skilled

SUMMARY

An individual's behavior is the result of a holistic process. This behavior is bounded by parameters of specific phenomena and is related to all other behaviors that occur at the same time. Program developers need a system for ordering behavioral objectives so as to provide for their interrelationships and expression in terms of directional progress goals.

A taxonomy of behavioral objectives, signifying a progressive development as determined by some organizing principle, provides a schema by which an objective can be placed on a continuum. Taxonomy facilitates communication among participants in the educational endeavor, clarifies the intended outcome, and promotes more acumen in evaluation.

Learning is expressed in three domains: cognitive, affective, and psychomotor. Although these three domains really are interdependent, development of a separate taxonomy for each is compatible with current teaching practices. This assures that all three domains receive equitable emphasis in the program and guides participants in the selection of appropriate learning experiences as well as in the development of suitable evaluation strategies. The use of open-ended behavioral objectives within the framework of the taxonomy enables faculty to focus the teaching–learning dynamic at the appropriate developmental level for any specific time in the program.

REFERENCES

American Nurses' Association. (1973). *Standards: Nursing practice.* Kansas City: Author.

American Nurses' Association. (1976). *Code for nurses with interpretative statements.* Kansas City: Author.

American Nurses' Association. (1980). *A social policy statement.* Kansas City: Author.

Benner, P., & Wrubel, J. (1989). *The primacy of caring: Stress and coping in health and illness.* Menlo Park, CA: Addison-Wesley.

Bloom, B. (Ed.). (1956). *Taxonomy of educational objectives, Handbook I: Cognitive domain.* New York: Longman.

Burton, M. R. (1976). *The influence of perceptual style and various combinations of mental and physical practice in facilitating the learning of a novel, fine complex perceptual-motor skill.* Unpublished doctoral dissertation, New York University.

Churchill, L. (1982). The teaching of ethics and moral values in teaching: Some contemporary confusions. *Journal of Higher Education, 53,* 296–306.

Cranston, M. (1983). Are there any human rights? *Daedalus, 112*(4), 1–18.

Dave, R. (1970). *Psychomotor levels in developing and writing objectives.* Tucson: Educational Innovators Press.

Davis, A., & Aroskar, M. (1983). *Ethical dilemmas and nursing practice* (2nd. ed.). Norwalk, CT: Appleton-Century-Crofts.

Dubos, R. (1981). *Celebration of life.* New York: McGraw-Hill.

Fleishman, E. (1972). A structure and measurement of psychomotor abilities. In R. Singer (Ed.), *The psychomotor domain: Movement behavior.* Philadelphia: Lea & Febiger.

Frankl, V. (1973). *Man's search for meaning.* New York: Washington Square Press.

Halpern, D. (1984). *Thought and knowledge.* Hillsdale, NJ: Lawrence Erlbaum Associates.

Hayter, J. (1983). Educational taxonomies revisited. *Journal of Nursing Education,* 22(8), 339–342.

Henry, F. (1958). Specificity vs generality in learning motor skills. *Proceedings of College Physical Education Association, 61,* 126–128.

Henry, W. (1990). Beyond the melting pot. *Time, 135*(15), 28–31.

Kelso, J. (Ed.). (1982). *Human motor behavior: An introduction.* Hillsdale, NJ: Lawrence Erlbaum Associates.

Kibler, R., Barker, L., & Miles, D. (1970). *Behavioral objectives and instruction.* Boston: Allyn & Bacon.

Kohlberg, L. (1981). *The philosophy of moral development.* New York: Harper & Row.

Krathwohl, D., Bloom, B., & Masia, B. (1964). *Taxonomy of educational objectives, Handbook II: Affective domain.* New York: Longman.

Marteniuk, R. (1969). Generality and specificity of learning and performance of two similar speed tasks. *Research Quarterly, 40,* 52.

Meyers, C. (1986). *Teaching students to think critically.* San Francisco: Jossey-Bass.

Miller, M. A., & Malcolm, N. S. (1990). Critical thinking in the nursing curriculum. *Nursing & Health Care, 11*(2), 67–73.

Oermann, M. H. (1991). *Professional nursing practice: A conceptual approach.* Philadelphia: J.B. Lippincott Co.

Podeschi, R. (1976). William James and education. *The Educational Forum, 40,* 223–229.

Raths, L., Harmin, M., & Simon, S. (1966). *Values and teaching.* Columbus, OH: Charles Merrill.

Reilly, D. (1989). Ethics and values in nursing: Are we opening Pandora's Box? *Nursing & Health Care, 10*(2), 91–95.

Reilly, D., & Oermann, M. (1985). *The clinical field: Its use in nursing education.* Norwalk, CT: Appleton-Century-Crofts.

Simpson, E. (1966). *The classification of educational objectives: Psychomotor domain.* Urbana, IL: University of Illinois Press.

Singer, R. (Ed.). (1975). *Motor learning and human performance.* New York: Macmillan.

Stent, G. (1977). The poverty of scientism and the promise of structuralist ethics. In H.T. Englehardt & D. Callahan (Eds.), *The foundation of ethics and its relationship to science, Vol 2, Knowledge, value and belief.* Hasting-on-the-Hudson, NY: Institute of Society, Ethics, and Life Sciences.

Tanner, D. (1972). *Using behavioral objectives in the classroom.* New York: Macmillan.

Tanner, C. A. (1983). Research on clinical judgment. In W.L. Holzemer (Ed.), *Review of research in nursing education* (pp. 2–32). Thorofare, NJ: Slack.

Tanner, C. A. (1987). Teaching clinical judgment. In J.J. Fitzpatrick & R.L. Taunton (Eds.), *Annual review of nursing research, Vol. 5* (pp. 153–173). New York: Springer.

Toulmin, S. (1977). The meaning of professionalism: Doctors, ethics, and biomedical science. In H.T. Erglehardt & D. Callahan (Eds.), *The foundation of ethics and its relationship to science, Vol 2, Knowledge, value and belief.* Hastings-On-the-Hudson, NY: Institute of Society, Ethics, and Life Sciences.

Watson, J. (1985). *Nursing: Human science and human care.* Norwalk, CT: Appleton-Century-Crofts.

Yinger, R. J. (1980). Can we really teach them to think? In R.E. Young (Ed.), *Fostering critical thinking.* San Francisco: Jossey-Bass.

RECOMMENDED READINGS

Aroskar, M. (1987). The interface of ethics and politics in nursing. *Nursing Outlook, 35*(6), 268–273.

Bandman, E. L., & Bandman, B. (1988). *Critical thinking in nursing.* Norwalk, CT: Appleton & Lange.

Benner, P., & Tanner, C. (1987). Clinical judgment: How expert nurses use intuition. *American Journal of Nursing, 87*(1), 23–31.

Benoliel, J. (1983). Ethics in nursing practice and education. *Nursing Outlook, 31,* 210–215.

Bonaparte, B. (1979). Ego defensiveness, open-closed mindness and nurses' attitudes toward culturally different patients. *Nursing Research, 28,* 166–171.

Brink, P. (1984). Value orientation as an assessment tool in cultural diversity. *Nursing Research, 33,* 198–203.

Cannon, R., Gilead, M., Haun, E., et al. (1984). A values clarification approach to cultural diversity. *Nursing & Health Care, 5,* 160–164.

Carnevali, D. L., Mitchell, P. H., Woods, N. F., & Tanner, C. A. (1984). *Diagnostic reasoning in nursing.* Philadelphia: J.B. Lippincott.

Dewey, J. (1975). *Moral principles in education.* Carbondale and Edwardsville, IL: Southern Illinois Press.

Dressler, D., Smejkal, C., & Ruffolo, M. (1983). A comparison of oral and rectal temperature measurement of patients receiving oxygen by mask. *Nursing Research, 32,* 373–375.

Eisenhauer, L. A., & Gendrop, S. (1990). Review of research on creative problem solving in nursing. In G.M. Glayton & P.A. Baj (Eds.), *Review of research in nursing education* (pp. 79–108). New York: National League for Nursing.

Elstein, A. S., Shulman, L. S., & Sprafka, S. A. (1978). *Medical problem-solving.* Cambridge: Harvard University Press.

Ethics in the academic profession. (1982). *Journal of Higher Education, 53.*

Field, P. A. (1987). The impact of nursing theory on the clinical decision making process. *Journal of Advanced Nursing, 12,* 563–571.

Frisch, N. (1987). Cognitive maturity of nursing students. *Image, 19*(1), 25–27.

Fromer, M. (1980). Teaching ethics by case conflicts. *Nursing Outlook, 28,* 604–608.

Fry, S. (1989). Toward a theory of nursing ethics. *Advances in Nursing Science, 11*(4), 9–22.

Gardner, J. (1978). *Morale.* New York: W.B. Saunders.

Gomez, G., & Gomez, E. (1987). Learning of psychiatric skills: laboratory vs patient care setting. *Journal of Nursing Education, 26*(1), 20–24.

Hannah, K. J., Reimer, M., Mills, W. C., & Letourneau, S. (Eds.). (1987). *Clinical judgment and decision making: The future with nursing diagnoses.* New York: John Wiley & Sons.

Harris, R. (1984). Clean vs. sterile tracheostomy care and level of pulmonary infection. *Nursing Research, 33,* 80–91.

Hilbert, G. (1985). Involvement of nursing students in unethical classroom and clinical behaviors. *Journal of Professional Nursing, 1*(4), 230–234.

Human Rights. (1983). *Daedalus, 112*(4).

Jones, J. A. (1988). Clinical reasoning in nursing. *Journal of Advanced Nursing, 13,* 185–192.

Johnson, D. (1984). *Computer ethics: A guide for the new age.* Elgin, IL: Brethen Press.

Kerr, R. (1982). *Psychomotor learning.* Philadelphia: Saunders.

Ketefian, S. (1981). Critical thinking, educational preparation and development of moral judgment among selected groups of practicing nurses. *Nursing Research, 30,* 98–103.

Kieffer, J. S. (1984). Selecting technical skills to teach for competency. *Journal of Nursing Education, 23*(5), 198–199.

Kitchener, K. S. (1983). Educational goals and reflective thinking. *Educational Forum, XLVII*(1), 75–79.

Kohlberg, L. (1978). The cognitive-development approach to moral education. In P. Scharf (Ed.), *Readings in moral education.* Minneapolis: Winston Press.

Larsen, D. (1983). *Computerized nursing skills simulations.* Philadelphia: Lippincott.

McInery, W. (1987). Understanding moral, issues in health care. *Journal of Professional Nursing, 3*(5), 268–277.

Mc Cormick, K. (1983). Preparing nurses for the technologic future. *Nursing & Health Care, 5,* 379–382.

Mooney, M. (1980). The ethical component of nursing theory: An analysis of ethical components in four nursing theories. *Image, 12*(1), 7–12.

Morrill, R. (1980). *Teaching values in college.* San Francisco: Jossey-Bass.

Munhall, P. (1980). Moral reasoning of nursing students and faculty in a baccalaureate program. *Image, 12*(3), 57–61.

Oermann, M. H. (1991). Psychomotor skill development. *Journal of Continuing Education in Nursing.*

Oxendine, J. (1984). *Psychology of motor learning* (2nd ed.). Englewood Cliffs, NJ: Prentice-Hall.

O'Rourke, K. (1983). Moral considerations in nursing curricula. *Journal of Nursing Education, 22,* 108–113.

Perry, W. (1970). *Forms of intellectual and ethical development in the college years.* New York: Holt, Rinehart & Winston.

Piaget, J. J. (1965). *The moral judgment of the child.* New York: Free Press.

Plunkett, E. J., & Olivieri, R. J. (1989). A strategy for introducing diagnostic reasoning: Hypothesis testing using a simulation approach. *Nurse Educator, 14*(6), 27–31.

Putzier, D. J., Padrick, K., Westfall, U. E., & Tanner, C. A. (1985). Diagnostic reasoning in critical care nursing. *Heart & Lung, 14*(5), 430–437.

Quinn, C., & Smith, N. (1987). *The professional commitment: Issues and ethics in nursing.* Philadelphia: W.B. Saunders.

Reilly, D. (1978). *Teaching and evaluating the affective domain in nursing programs.* Thorofare, NJ: Charles B. Slack.

Scheibe, K. (1970). *Beliefs and values.* New York: Holt, Rinehart & Winston.

Schein, E. (1972). *Professional education: Some new directions.* New York: McGraw-Hill.

Schneider, W., & Fish, A. (1982). Attention theory and mechanisms for skilled performance. *ERIC Reports,* Champagne, IL: Illinois University.

Steele, S., & Harmon, V. (1983). *Values clarification in nursing* (2nd ed.). Norwalk, CT: Appleton-Century-Crofts.

Stelmach, G. (1978). *Information processing and motor control learning.* New York: Academic Press.

Sweeney, M., Regan, P., O'Malley, M., & Hedstrom, B. (1980). Essential skills for baccalaureate graduates: Perspectives of education and service. *Journal of Administration, 10,* 37–44.

Tanner, C. A., Padrick, K. P., Westfall, U. E., & Putzier, D. J. (1987). Diagnostic reasoning strategies of nurses and nursing students. *Nursing Research, 36*(6), 358–363.

Thompson, K. (1981). Changes in the values and life styles preferences of university students. *Journal of Higher Education, 52,* 506–518.

5

Systematic Approach to the Development of Behavioral Objectives in a Nursing Program

As has been previously stated, a behavioral objective or a set of behavioral objectives does not exist in a vacuum, but is always part of a larger system. Within the larger system such objectives contribute to its viability and in turn derive vitality from it.

A systems approach to educational programs is not new to nursing. Following the medical model, nursing programs developed around body systems, and nursing care was taught as specifically related to each system. Modern systems theories directed nursing into a search for a systems model that is more representative of nursing practice. Chin (1961) refers to a conceptual model of practice when he states, "All practitioners have ways of thinking about and figuring out situations of change. These ways are embedded in the concepts with which they apprehend the dynamics of the client system they are working with, their relationship to it, and their process of helping with the change" (p. 201).

It is not within the scope of this book to present conceptual models for nursing or for nursing education. This chapter, however, does demonstrate a systematic approach to the evolution of behavioral objectives within a nursing education program which promotes an educational rather than a training program.

DEVELOPMENTAL MODEL

A system may be conceptualized as a phenomenon, a gestalt, composed of parts or elements, and as connected to each other so that interaction, interdependence, and integration occur. Boundaries of a particular system represent a closure around selected variables of the phenomenon, so that the energy exchange occurs primarily within the closure and little occurs between the system and its outside environs. Parts of the system may be referred to as subsystems, each with its own structure and function and a certain degree of autonomy. Each subsystem has its own goals and energy for self maintenance, growth, and self perpetuation. It is open and connected to other subsystems, and thus is susceptible to a disturbance in other parts of the subsystem.

Chin's developmental model is compatible with the concept of education as a force expediting the development of human potential. Chin (1961) characterizes the developmental model in the following manner:

> By developmental models, we mean those bodies of thought that center around growth and directional change. Developmental models assume change; they assume that there are noticeable differences between the states of a system at different times; that the succession of these states implies the system is heading somewhere; and that there are orderly processes which explain how the system gets from its present state to where it is going (p. 208).

In this model, one may refer to stages rather than to subsystems, but each stage can be identified and each meets the characteristics described for subsystems. With this model the learner's growth and development become critical variables, and behavioral objectives are expressed in terms of directional progress goals. Since the taxonomies, as described in previous chapters, are also predicated on the assumption that growth in each of the three domains (cognitive, affective, and psychomotor) is the main goal of educational endeavors, the taxonomies provide a methodology for the developmental model of behavioral objectives.

SYSTEMS MODEL FOR NURSING CURRICULUM

Why use a system model approach to curriculum development in nursing education? Professional programs of study, unlike some liberal arts fields, are sequential and progressive, that is, each experiences draws on previous experiences and is foundational to the next experience. Bruner (1973), a recognized educational theorist, believes that teaching the structure of a subject is the essential element in education. He describes learning the structure of a subject so as to understand it in a way that permits many other things to be related to it meaningfully (p. 7). Knowledge of the structure of a subject facilitates its transfer to more complex phenomena. Bruner suggests a spiral curriculum whereby, once the structure of a subject is learned, it is related to increasingly complex phenomena. A spiral curriculum in nursing education implies the student learning the basic structure of nursing and then, through increasingly complex encounters with nursing phenomena, a gestalt of nursing evolves which is compatible with a professional concept.

Such an evolution suggests an orderly process whereby a deliberate protocol for increasing the complexity of student experience with nursing exists. Bruner (1966) perceives curriculum as involving mastery of skills that in turn lead to mastery of more powerful skills, the establishment of self-received sequences.

A system approach to curriculum development—providing order, direction, and structure—is compatible with the concept of a spiral curriculum. It provides a common frame of reference for the many instructors involved in a nursing program, each with unique abilities and foci of interest, so that all would be contributing toward attainment of outcomes agreed on by faculty. Bevis (1989) notes the significance of course, unit, modules, and/or learning activities objectives as building blocks toward the attainment of program objectives derived from the conceptual framework.

Is such a structural approach stifling to the potential creativity of learners and teachers and a deterrent to accommodating new concepts, ideas, and experiences? Tyler (1950) proposed a way of systemizing curriculum development; framework, program objectives, course, and level objectives which would be translated into learning experiences and evaluation strategies. Since the behavioral objectives he proposed were open-ended and not stated in behavioral terms that could be measured or observed, they were not derived from behaviorism theory. His proposal, therefore, provides opportunity for teaching-learning experiences to be truly transformational. Bevis and Clayton (1988) see such a system approach as providing a prescriptive, rule-driven curriculum and question whether its products can "provide the impetus for the creative, individualized context-responsive, caring, human-services-oriented, humanistic, critical thinking, human science education that should form the basis for nursing" (p. 15).

Throughout this text, the position of the authors is that structure does not necessarily imply restrictive control, especially if humanistic sciences influence the preparation of behavioral objectives and their translation into teaching-learning situations and evaluation. Rather than rule-driven, such a curriculum would be logic-driven. When a rule-driven curriculum exists, it is often the function of the individuals responsible for administering and teaching in it who tend to be more comfortable when controlling events then when risking new experiences. But a rule-driven curriculum is not necessarily related to the notion of a system-directed curriculum.

The use of a system approach is presented here with samples of open-ended objectives and potential behaviors that relate to each objective. It is, of course, the perogative of each instructor to delineate the particular behaviors for each of the objectives which provide direction for assessing the student's mastery of the objective. Such action helps faculty to develop a focus which is fair for all learners and enables the student to have some frame of reference for developing the learning implied in the objective. As in any human science endeavor, such behaviors should not be treated as absolutes and accommodations must be provided for those additional behaviors that are significant to the situation or unique to the learner.

APPLICATION OF SYSTEMS MODEL
IN NURSING EDUCATION PROGRAMS

For our present purposes, it can be said that the system involves behavioral objectives of the program as well as all stages or subsystems of the program related to objectives. It is important to remind the reader, however, that the derivation of the program of behavioral objectives results from an exploration of seven areas; nature of person, societal trends and goals, professional issues and trends, nature of the learner, concept of the teaching–learning process, philosophy of the agency offering the program, and models of nursing.

The system of the program for the school of nursing would include subsystems of behavioral objectives, as shown in the Systems Model of Program Behavioral Objectives (Fig. 5–1).

Program behavioral objectives are those a faculty and other participants in program planning determine as desirable outcomes. In some instances these objectives are referred to as *terminal* objectives. The word *terminal*, however, carries a connotation of finality inconsistent with concepts of continuity in development and life-long learning. The term *outcome*, which the authors of this book favor, has a more dynamic quality.

Level behavioral objectives are those expected of a learner at a particular point in time in the program. The time dimension may be defined in terms of years in a program, completion of a certain group of courses or learning experiences, or period in which an individual has reached a designated level of

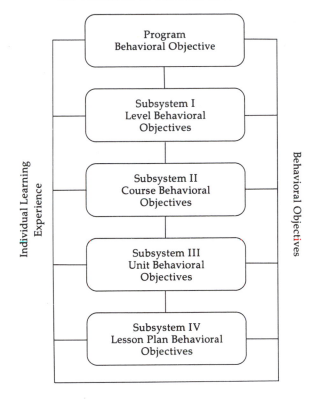

Figure 5-1
Systems Model of Program Behavioral Objectives

competency. Since learning is perceived as a developmental process, levels should not occur at too frequent intervals; this would ensure that sufficient time is allowed for change.

Course behavioral objectives are outcomes expected at the conclusion of the course. If the course is divided into units, then behavioral objectives are expressed for each unit. If the nurse teacher uses individual lesson plans, then appropriate behavioral objectives are identified. Behavioral objectives for individual learning experiences may be chosen to flow from any of the subsystems or directly from the program behavior objective depicted in Figure 5-1.

Modifications in the model will be made for continuing education or for in-service education programs. Program behavioral objectives would, of course, be the initial stage. Level behavioral objectives exist if the program is based within a developmental context identifiable in stages. Course behavioral objectives come into consideration if courses or unified blocks of learning are designed for the program. Inclusion of unit behavioral objectives depends on the organization of the program. Lesson plan and individual learning experience behavioral objectives are similar in development to those suggested for nursing programs in schools of nursing.

INTERRELATIONSHIP OF SUBSYSTEMS OF BEHAVIORAL OBJECTIVES

The Systems Model of Program Behavioral Objectives (Fig. 5–1) connotes an interrelationship among subsystems of behavioral objectives; yet, in too many instances each subsystem is treated as a separate entity. Each subsystem of behavioral objectives meets the criteria of a subsystem; each has its own structure and functions with a certain degree of autonomy and demonstrates the energy for self-maintenance, growth, and self-perpetuation. However, other criteria—open and connected to other subsystems—seem to be ignored by many nurse teachers, with autonomy of the subsystem being given primary consideration. If, within a system, all subsystems contribute to each other and to the totality of the system, then all subsystems of behavioral objectives must be interrelated. Individuals responsible for planning behavioral objectives at each level do not have complete autonomy; rather, they must be certain that their planning is consistent with that of other parts of the system.

Program development moves from general to specific; that is, program behavioral objectives are determined first. Then, using a developmental concept, level behavioral outcomes are defined. The number of levels depends on their definition as described by the planners. The final level and program behavioral objectives are the same; for example, behavioral objectives for the senior year of a baccalaureate program are the same as program behavioral objectives since it is assumed that the learner will meet criteria for the latter by the end of the program.

Planners determine the framework for courses within each level, and behavioral objectives for each course are written accordingly. If a level represents a considerable time span, such as a year in a nursing program, it must be remembered that the planners perceived that period of time as essential for most learners to achieve the competency described. Therefore, behavioral objectives for courses that terminate earlier in the term would be at a lower developmental level. Single behaviors identified primarily with a course, such as skill in listening to a fetal heart, are defined according to the expectation of faculty involved and not constrained by behavioral objectives at a given level.

Unit behavioral objectives are derived from course behavioral objectives, and lesson plan behavioral objectives are derived from unit behavioral objectives. Individual learning experience behavioral objectives vary in their source, arising from behavioral objectives for any part of the system.

The process of producing behavioral objectives within this system utilizes the Chin developmental model as a framework, and the taxonomies as the method for identifying behaviors in each stage of development.

INTERDOMAIN BEHAVIORS

Before demonstrating the process, more needs to be said about behavioral objectives as written for each subsystem. As stated previously, a behavior is multidimensional, often involves two or more domains of learning, and is a composite of a series of behaviors. The domain selected as the primary focus of the behavioral objective is a judgment made by the planners, but behaviors that comprise a behavioral objective may represent all domains. Therefore when behavioral objectives for any of the stages are written, they must include the composite of behaviors from the various domains accepted as evidence of achievement of the objective. The behaviors also bring into sharp focus those methodologies and learning experiences relevant to the behavioral objective.

Development within each domain of learning is independent of that which occurs in the other domains. That is, the achievement of the analytic level in the cognitive domain at 4.1 does not necessarily mean that an affective domain behavior within the objective will also be at the 4.1 level in that domain. There must be a reasonable relationship of levels among behaviors, but each domain behavior must be treated as a discrete entity.

Following is a behavioral objective with its components for data analysis in the nursing process. It is at the level expected of a practitioner.*

BEHAVIORAL OBJECTIVE

At the end of the course, the nursing student will

C4.2   Relate concepts of self-care to nursing management of clients with chronic pain.

BEHAVIORS

C4.2   Analyzes the relationship between theories of pain and concepts of self-care.

* The 'C' before the behavior means cognitive domain; the 'A' means affective domain; and the 'P' means psychomotor domain.

C4.2   Appraises the biopsychosocial and cultural influences on the individual's ability to manage own pain.

C4.2   Identifies the impact of chronic pain on the developmental tasks of the client.

C4.2   Analyzes the impact of chronic pain on family relationships and dynamics.

C4.2   Identifies scientific rationale underlying traditional and nontraditional methods of chronic pain management.

C4.2   Identifies criteria for distinguishing between use of traditional and nontraditional methods of pain management.

A4.1   Defends the client's right to be informed regarding traditional and nontraditional methods of chronic pain management.

C4.2   Analyzes nontraditional methods of pain management in terms of the client's and family's learning needs and self-care potential.

A3.3   Supports the client's choice regarding the selection of methods for pain management.

In the above example, the behavioral objective is identified within the cognitive domain at the analytic level, according to the taxonomy. Nine behaviors, representative of affective and cognitive domains, are described for this behavioral objective. In this illustration, the psychomotor domain is not relevant. The level ascribed to the behavioral objective would be expected of a senior student in a professional program or a professional practitioner. Behaviors of the domain identified in the behavioral objective are generally expressed within the same level as the objective; although there may be reasons that lead faculty to expect students to reach a higher or lower level of competency in a particular behavior.

Not only may behaviors within a behavioral objective represent different domains of learning, but so, too, may the development of behavioral objectives, or behaviors listed under the objective, change in domain as they progress through the system. In the discussion of affective behaviors, it was noted that cognition is an important part of the valuing process. Thus, in the development of values, behaviors may first be expressed in the affective domain, then in the cognitive domain, and once again in the affective domain. Using an affective behavior, the development process in a nursing program with three levels would be:

Level I   A2.2   The nursing student discusses willingly the rights of clients to be informed regarding health problems and management.

Level II   C3.0   The nursing student examines traditional and nontraditional methods of pain management risks and outcomes from a scientific basis.

Level III   A3.3   The nursing student accepts responsibility for assuring that the client is knowledgeable about differences between traditional and nontraditional chronic pain therapies.

In some instances, the development of affective behavior may move from cognitive to affective domains through several levels of the affective taxonomy.

Level I   C2.3   The nursing student differentiates between traditional and nontraditional methods of chronic pain management in terms of scientific action.

Level II   A3.3   The nursing student assumes responsibility for informing the client about both traditional and nontraditional methods of chronic pain management.

Level III   A4.1   The nursing student defends the client's right to be informed regarding traditional and nontraditional methods of chronic pain management.

The Level III behavior in this illustration is determined by the planner, as the expected outcome. Then judgments are made as to whether the cognitive or affective domain is to be the focal point. The decision may well be that all three levels are in the affective domain.

Likewise, a cognitive behavior may not begin in the cognitive domain but in the affective domain instead:

Level I   A2.3   The nursing student takes the initiative in seeking readings that increase the understanding of various sociocultural interpretations of the concepts of health and illness.

Level II   C3.0   The nursing student uses relevant sociocultural concepts of health and illness in assessing the health needs of a particular patient and family.

Level III   C4.2   The nursing student relates the patient's response to health or illness to sociocultural background.

Cognitive behaviors also may be developed only within the one domain, the cognitive.

AFFECTIVE OBJECTIVES AND BEHAVIORS

The following are examples of affective behavioral objectives and their behaviors.

BEHAVIORAL OBJECTIVE

A3.1   The student provides opportunity for the hospitalized adult to express own beliefs, interests, and needs.

BEHAVIORS

A3.1   Accepts responsibility for listening to clients express ideas for plans of care

A3.1   Encourages client to express own concerns

A3.1   Considers client's preferences when they are supportive of his or her care

C3.0   Makes adjustments in nursing care to meet expressed needs of the client

A3.1   Supports the client's right to confidentiality

BEHAVIORAL OBJECTIVE

A3.2   The student accepts responsibility for developing competence in carrying out a psychosocial assessment process

BEHAVIORS

C3.0   Identifies personal variables which influence the psychosocial assessment

C2.3   Determines own response to clients of varied cultural, religious, and sexual life styles

A3.2   Examines willingly own feelings about the data obtained in a psychosocial assessment process

A3.2   Discusses with other nursing colleagues own feelings and actions regarding the psychosocial assessment process

A3.2   Assumes responsibility for reviewing the literature and current research relating to psychosocial assessment

A3.2   Assumes responsibility for self-direction in obtaining assessment experiences as needed for reaching competency

THE DEVELOPMENTAL PROCESS
IN RELATION TO OBJECTIVES

Behaviors are developed progressively throughout the nursing program; this development is reflected in the objectives which depict movement of the learner through the system. The sequencing or leveling of objectives begins with determining the program objectives which indicate the outcomes expected at the end of the program. The program and the senior year objective are identical since the program objective is to be achieved at the conclusion of the senior year. Based on the number of levels in the curriculum, a level being a particular point in time such as the sophomore year, objectives are written at each level. Course objectives represent the outcomes expected at the conclusion of a course. Some courses are divided into units and specify objectives for achievement at the completion of the unit. For faculty who develop lesson plans, objectives derived from the unit objectives may be written to indicate the learning outcomes at the end of a particular lesson.

Table 5–1 illustrates the process of sequencing objectives in a baccalaureate nursing program from the program objective through individual behaviors within a course in the sophomore year. The ultimate level of learning, reflected in the program objective, is at the analysis level. In the junior year, the focus is on using the nursing process with individual clients and families of varying ages and with different types of health problems. Courses in the junior year, then, provide experiences with both individuals and families throughout the life cycle; multiple types of health problems can be addressed. In the sophomore year, learning outcome relates to demonstrating use of the nursing process with individual clients only. At this level there is an understanding of the nursing process but direction is needed in carrying it out in the clinical field. Courses and their units within the sophomore year contribute to the development of this ability. The illustration also includes a related unit objective and individual behaviors that the student must meet to demonstrate that the unit objective has been achieved.

An important point in this illustration is that all parts of the system contribute to achieving the program objective. Unit objectives are derived from course objectives, course from level objectives, and level from program objectives.

Table 5–2 shows a similar process of development for an associate degree of diploma nursing program. The program objective represents use of the nursing process with clients and families in multiple settings. Generally, in these programs there are two levels. The second level and the program objective are

Table 5–1
Behavioral Objectives Sequence—
Program to Unit—Baccalaureate Program

System	Program (Senior Level)	C4.2	The nursing student uses the nursing process in meeting the health care needs of individuals, families, and groups.
Subsystem I	Junior Level	C3.0	The nursing student uses the nursing process in meeting the health care needs of individuals and families throughout the life cycle with varying health problems.
	Sophomore Level	C2.2	The nursing student demonstrates use of the nursing process in meeting the health needs of individuals.
Subsystem II	Course: Concepts Basic to Professional Nursing Practice	C2.2	The nursing student relates various theoretical concepts to the nursing process.
Subsystem III	Unit: Nursing Process	C2.2	The nursing student describes the nursing process and its relationship to meeting the health care needs of clients.
	Unit Behaviors	C2.2	Describes stages of the nursing process and their interrelationship.
		C2.2	Explains the relationship of the nursing process to meeting individual health care needs.
		A2.2	Discusses willingly the impact of the nurse's own biases and values in the various stages of the nursing process.
		C2.2	Interprets the relationship among assessment, nursing diagnoses, and plan of care.
		C2.2	Describes the purpose of the evaluation stage of the nursing process.

Table 5–2
Behavioral Objectives Sequence—Program to Unit—
Associate Degree or Diploma Program (Two Years)

System	Program (Second Level)	C3.0	The nursing student uses the nursing process in meeting the health needs of clients and families in varied settings.
Subsystem I	First Level	C2.2	The nursing student demonstrates use of the nursing process in meeting the health needs of adult patients.
Subsystem II	Course: Care of Adults with Chronic Health Problems	C2.2	The nursing student demonstrates use of the nursing process with care of adults with chronic health problems.
Subsystem III	Unit: Nursing Process	C2.2	The nursing student demonstrates use of the nursing process in meeting the needs of aged patients with chronic health problems.
	Unit Behaviors	C2.2	Assesses needs of aged patients with chronic health problems.
		P3.0	Takes accurately vital signs within the assessment process.
		C2.2	Gives examples of nursing diagnosis for clients with selected chronic health problems.
		C2.2	Develops plan of care considering chronicity of illness.
		C2.2	Implements established plan of care including referrals to other health care professionals.
		A2.2	Discusses willingly own feelings and values regarding care of an adult with a chronic illness.

identical. The first level objective, which is at the comprehension level, indicates use of the nursing process with supervision; courses within this particular level focus on care of adults only. The course objective, Care of Adults with Chronic Health Problems, is also at the comprehension level. The unit objective indicates that this particular course is divided into units, one of which pertains to the use of the nursing process with aged persons. The behaviors for the unit which the student is expected to attain are identified.

Both illustrations suggest a systematic approach to the development of behavioral objectives which combines the developmental model with use of the taxonomies. This process provides a means of sequencing objectives throughout a nursing program to reflect the progressive development of knowledge, skills, and values.

The levels identified with staff development and continuing education programs depend on the framework in which they are defined. The process for developing objectives is the same as described here since behaviors still need to be developed in a progressive manner.

USE OF SYSTEMS MODEL
FOR LEVELING OBJECTIVES

The Systems Model (Fig. 5–1), based on Chin's developmental model, assumes that nursing education is a developmental process identifiable by specifically defined levels. A level is a point in the development scale which defines certain competencies to be achieved and demands that the teacher and learner be accountable for their attainment. If attainment has not been achieved, then a rationale must be provided from supporting data.

The use of the model implies that in a nursing education program, the learner's growth and development in relation to the competencies needed of a nurse practitioner become the critical variables in the program. The competencies defined as behavioral outcomes at each level are expressed in terms of directional progress goals, for all levels must ultimately contribute to the program objectives as defined by the faculty of a program.

It is essential that the program outcomes be realistic within the framework of the present educational system and the resources available to the faculty. Argyris and Schön (1974) warn us that "the school cannot claim the entire function of helping students to acquire professional competence—at least not without restructuring the concepts of school and office so that the traditional boundaries between them virtually disappear." As they address the incompatibilities between the time and experiences needed to develop professional competencies and the structure of school experiences such as course work, term papers, defined school terms, etc., they remind us that the intensity and duration of involvement in practice are too limited in educational programs to enable the student to acquire a full range of professional competence (p. 186).

Program objectives are general objectives which encompass behaviors in all domains: cognitive, affective, and psychomotor. The objectives are stated as outcomes (some people call these objectives *terminal*) and then specific behaviors are developed under each objective. These behaviors indicate what the student must accomplish in order to demonstrate attainment of the objective.

The delineation of program objectives for a nursing program is dependent on the concept of nursing accepted by a faculty. Nursing, as perceived by the authors, is a theoretically derived practice discipline based on a value system reflective of the inherent worth and dignity of an individual. This concept then suggests six possible areas which must be reflected in a set of program objectives of a nursing education program.

1. *Theory framework* of the curriculum, such as: adaptation, caring, needs, self-care, behavior systems, life process.

   EXAMPLE: The student practices nursing within the adaptation framework as it relates to the client in all stages of development at any point on the health-illness continuum.

2. *Nursing methodology* —nursing process.

   EXAMPLE: The student uses the nursing process in meeting the health care needs of clients.

3. *Concept of inherent worth and dignity of the individual* —may be stated as an objective or may be combined with another objective.

   EXAMPLE: The student accepts responsibility to provide nursing care reflective of an individual client's inherent worth and dignity.

4. *Interrelationships* —often refers to intra- and inter-disciplinary interactions; may also refer to client interactions.

   EXAMPLE: The student interacts in a facilitative, purposeful manner with clients, families, colleagues, and members of other health care disciplines.

5. *Student development* —toward self actualization.

   EXAMPLE: The student develops a self-identity which supports continued development as a learner, nursing practitioner, and a contributing member of society.

6. *Profession* —relates to the practitioner and the profession as they interface with the health of society and patterns of health care organization.

   EXAMPLE: The student identifies the dimensions of accountability of the nurse and the profession toward society as they seek to meet the health care needs of their constituents.

7. *Research*—may be included as a separate objective in baccalaureate and higher degree programs which have development of research competencies as a outcome of the program.

EXAMPLE: The student applies findings of nursing and other health-related research in practice.

These areas represent, for the most part, the dimensions of a basic program toward which development should be directed. It is important that not too many objectives be stated, for once the objectives become too specific, there is the real danger of exclusion of other equitable behaviors—that is, inclusion can often lead to exclusion. The behavioral level at which these objectives are designated and the complexity of variables with which these behaviors occur are determined by the type of educational program for which they have been developed.

Once the faculty has prepared the outcome objectives, they are leveled to indicate the progression in their development. The number of levels in a program is determined by the faculty. Many use years in a program as a framework for identifying levels. Levels must be of sufficient length of time for learning to occur, therefore, they should be limited in number for any particular educational program.

There are two ways in which leveling of objectives may be accomplished. The behavior itself may be changed to indicate a higher taxonomy level or the variables with which the behavior is to be carried out may be changed to indicate complexity. The ability to use the nursing process is more complex (i.e., higher level) than the ability to explain the nursing process. Likewise, the skills used in the nursing process with individuals are less complex than those used with groups.

With some leveling, only the behavior is changed; with others only the variables concerned with the behavior are altered; whereas in some instances both the behavior and variables are changed.

EXAMPLE: *Level I*

The student *explains* the nursing process as it relates to the care of a *patient*.

EXAMPLE: *Level II*

The student *uses* the nursing process to provide care to *the patient and his family*.

Leveling thus first involves the delineation of objectives as outcomes for the program. It is important to remember that since these objectives state the competencies expected at the conclusion of the program, they must be attainable and measurable. Therefore, they should not represent a projection of what the student will achieve as a graduate. The objectives cannot state an expectation that the student will be accountable for nursing practice as a professional nurse. The student, at the program's conclusion, is not a professional nurse. That behavior must be evaluated at a later time in a study of graduates.

It is also important to recognize that the objectives of the program are also the objectives of the last year of the program. If the objectives define expectations of competency at the conclusion of the program, that conclusion occurs at the end of the last year. There is no need for senior-level objectives in a program; they are already stated.

After these program objectives have been developed, the behaviors for each objective must be stated. These behaviors indicate the specific behaviors that the student will demonstrate to validate achievement of the objective. These behaviors also are subject to the leveling process.

SUMMARY

A systematic approach to the development of behavioral objectives is predicated on the assumption that a system (program behavioral objectives) exists in which subsystems are included, namely, level, course, unit, behavioral objectives as well as lesson or individual learning experience objectives. The system model is relevant to a professional educational curriculum which is sequential and progressive. It provides a framework when used with a taxonomy for expressing learning outcomes at various stages in the program within a developmental context. The systems model assures the continuity and interrelationship of the various levels in the curriculum so that all levels contribute to the outcomes stated for the program. As with any system, however, professional judgment is always important for making accommodations for the special needs and abilities of individual students.

REFERENCES

Argyris, C., & Schön, D. (1974). *Theory in practice: Increasing professional effectiveness.* San Francisco: Jossey-Bass.

Bevis, E. (1989). *Curriculum building in nursing: A process* (3rd ed.). New York: National League for Nursing.

Bevis, E., & Clayton, G. (1988). Needed: A new curriculum development design. *Nurse Educator, 13*(4), 14–17.

Bruner, J. (1963). *The process of education.* New York: Vintage Books.

Bruner, J. (1966). *Toward a theory of instruction.* Cambridge: Belknap Press of Harvard University Press.

Chin, R. (1961). The utility of systems models and developmental models for practitioners. In W. Bennis, K. Benne, & R. Chin (Eds.), *The planning of change.* New York: Holt, Rinehart & Winston.

Tyler, R. (1950). *Basic principles of curriculum and instruction.* Chicago: University of Chicago Press.

RECOMMENDED READINGS

Bloom, B. (Ed.). (1956). *Taxonomy of behavioral objectives: Handbook I: Cognitive domain.* New York: Longman.

Conrad, C., & Pratt, A. (1983). Making decisions about the curriculum. *Journal of Higher Education, 54,* 15–30.

Diekelmann, N. (1989). The nursing curriculum: Lived experiences of students. In *Curriculum revolution: Reconceptualizing nursing education* (pp. 25–42). New York: National League for Nursing.

Hunkins, F. (1980). *Curriculum development: Program improvement.* Columbus, OH: Charles Merrill.

King, I. (1986). *Curriculum and instruction in nursing.* Norwalk, CT: Appleton-Century-Crofts.

Krathwohl, D., Bloom, B., & Masia, B. (1964). *Taxonomy of educational objectives: Handbook II: Affective domain.* New York: Longman.

Lawrence, S., & Lawrence, R. (1983). Curriculum development: Philosophy, objectives, and conceptual framework. *Nursing Outlook, 31,* 160–163.

Reilly, C., & Oermann, M. (1985). *The clinical field: Its use in nursing education.* Norwalk, CT: Appleton-Century-Crofts.

Smith, C. (1984). Process curriculum in nursing contrasted to product orientation. *Journal of Nursing Education, 23,* 167–169.

Van Ort, S., & Putt, A. (1985). *Teaching in collegiate schools of nursing.* Boston: Little, Brown & Co.

6

Preparation of Behavioral Objectives for Continuing Education or Staff Development Programs

The preparation of behavioral objectives for continuing education and staff development programs occurs within a framework which is similar to, but also different from, that of the more formalized programs of study in a nursing school. For the most part, behavioral objectives for these programs are directed toward a narrow, specific area of nursing knowledge or practice offered within a short span of time. The technique of writing these behavioral objectives is the same as for all educational programs, but the limiting characteristic of continuing education and staff development programs challenges the program planner in relation to substance and outcome expectations.

In this chapter, the term *continuing education program* encompasses the concept of staff development programs. It is recognized that some nurse educators differentiate between these two types of programs, but a definition of a continuing education program which refers to an education program directed toward the learning needs of practitioners would also include staff development programs.

BEHAVIORAL OBJECTIVES AS A CONTRACT

The statement of objectives for a continuing education program is in essence a contract with the consumer, for it tells the individual what is the expected outcome of that experience. The statement is one of the most important factors in influencing a consumer to participate in the program.

The increasing demand for continuing education programs to meet the needs of practitioners who must continuously update knowledge and practice competencies challenges program planners to develop programs that are relevant, worthwhile, and of high quality. Reilly (1976) states: "The institution of a requirement such as continuing education places demands upon constituents, employees, and the public. These demands are economic, social, temporal, intellectual, physical, and emotional. Because of the multifaceted nature of these demands, it is most important that program planners assure that their offerings merit the expenditures entailed" (p. 30). Behavioral objectives stated clearly so as to define the focus of the program and a program plan consistent with the stated objectives must be communicated to the target population so that the membership will be informed as to what it is purchasing. Objectives are a significant component of continuing education programs. They are not a pedagogical exercise representing a skill in combining words and phrases into some fine sounding statement reflective of current fads in educational or nursing jargon. They are, instead, reflective statements of what is to be and must meet the test of "truth in advertising" demanded by consumers in all parts of our society. They communicate the intent and direction of the program and require the program planners to be held accountable for providing opportunities for the participants to obtain the objectives.

The statement of behavioral objectives does not guarantee that all participants will attain the objectives, for the achievement of any individual rests with that person's readiness and motivation to learn. The program planner is stating, however, that there will be opportunity provided to engage in the specified learning. The stated objectives enable the individual to have the knowledge of the learning to be achieved and the option to make the decision as to whether or not that learning is wanted or needed.

PURPOSE OF CONTINUING EDUCATION PROGRAMS

What is the goal of all continuing education programs in nursing? The position of the continuing educator is found within professional schools and health care agencies. The early stages in the development of such a position in health care agencies provided solely for instruction in orientation of new personnel or on-the-job training for certain classifications of personnel. Universities and other institutions of higher learning focused their energies on moving nurses through the academic route with a degree as the sign of achievement. Although there were great pronouncements about the expanding knowledge base of nursing practice as new developments occurred in its related science fields, little emphasis was given to the need of the nurse in practice to update knowledge and competencies. When the need was recognized, many nursing continuing education programs followed the historical route and sought assistance from people outside the discipline. Thus many programs were provided by doctors, pharmacists, educationists, psychologists, etc. Very few program planners called on members of the nursing discipline to help the nurse broaden knowledge and competencies that led to greater depth in nursing practice. It was also noted that while nursing has called on these outside disciplines, nursing has not been asked to contribute to knowledge of the practitioners in those disciplines. The interdisciplinary teaching was unilateral.

These comments are not intended to suggest that all programs must be conducted by nurses: they are to suggest that a nursing educator's business is to assist with the practitioner's practice and that the contribution of various disciplines must be seen within that context.

The goal of continuing education programs must relate to the nature of the nursing discipline. Nursing is a theoretically based practice discipline based on a value system reflective of man's inherent dignity and worth. What does this conceptualization of practice suggest to the program planners about the substance of the objectives they develop? It certainly identifies the nurse practitioner as a user of knowledge, especially as the profession is now developing its own generators of knowledge, the nurse researchers. However, most of the programs offered are geared toward the in-depth preparation of the nurse as a user of knowledge by expanding the theory base and by helping with the development of problem solving and decision making skills. Varied assessment and intervention competencies are also legitimate concerns of continuing education programs.

SOURCES OF BEHAVIORAL OBJECTIVES

The critical question in the preparation of behavioral objectives for a program relates to the WHAT, the substance of the objectives. Where does one go to find the focus in order to be able to select the appropriate outcomes that are relevant to the target population for whom the program is designed?

There are four areas where competency is expected of any nurse practitioner today. These areas provide an excellent source for identifying the content of any continuing education offering.

1. *A nursing model as a framework for practice.* This area is a rapidly evolving dimension in nursing and is a critical one if nursing is to define its own limits of practice. Theory development in nursing is making rapid strides toward an eventual nursing science. Currently, nursing practice is moving within conceptual frameworks that describe nursing practice rather than predict it as a theory could. These frameworks are directed toward helping nurses view their practice from a nursing perspective rather than from a medical model. What are continuing educators doing to help the nurse in practice understand the theory behind practice and the evolution of a nursing model? Is this information to be maintained only for the new practitioners and the graduate prepared nurses located in universities? Do not current practitioners also need this new knowledge to impact their own actions?

2. *Nursing process.* This second area relates to the way one nurses. It addresses nursing's method of practice. It states that nursing is a problem-solving process demanding decision making and clinical judgment rather than being a task-oriented discipline as many perceive it to be. The process incorporates skills in data gathering, scientific interpretation, nursing diagnoses, intervention, and finally evaluation for determining both the outcome of care and the process by which the nurse arrived at the outcome. Every profession has its own method of operation. Nursing process is nursing's method. It represents all domains of action—cognitive, affective, psychomotor—within a moral and ethical framework. Continuing education programs need to focus on skill development in nursing process. Emphasis in programs on one aspect, such as physical assessment skills, without relating these skills to all other aspects of the process perpetuate the task approach to nursing.

3. *Interpersonal skills.* Nurses are in the people business. Competency in interacting with clients, families, colleagues, other disciplines, and the public is essential if nursing actions are to be effective. This area incorporates many focal points for evolving programs. The various theories, concepts, and processes as well as techniques and strategies are all legitimate areas of concern.

4. *Membership in a profession.* This area is concerned with the responsibilities inherent in membership in a collective group—a profession. Concerns here relate not only to the nurse's own role but to the role of a profession within a worldwide community. Nursing practice is developed and functions within a professional framework. The focus of the behavioral objectives must also be relevant to that framework, especially in terms of the trends, movements, and future goals of that profession. The changing role of the nurse as newer health needs emerge, the interface of nursing with other health related disciplines, the empowerment of nursing, the economics of health care pertinent to payment for nursing services, issues about quality assurance programs for care, the legislative actions which relate to nursing practice and nursing education, and the credentialing of nursing's educational programs and services are all legitimate areas for the development of objectives.

Objectives must also reflect the issues, movements, and concerns of the society to which we belong. Although our professional sphere occupies a considerable portion of our life, neither that profession nor we as individuals live in a vacuum. We are constantly interfacing with many facets of our society and the clients we serve are of that society. Therefore, as behavioral objectives are prepared, they must reflect the real world. What are the implications of biases based on race, religion, sex, physical deformities, and age on the nurse's approach to the clients? What do inflation, violence, changing nature of family structure, consumer movements, and environmental issues have to do with the programs offered? Outcomes must be designed to help the nurse live and work within a changing society, where the absolutes of good and bad no longer apply with the certainty that many older practitioners remember. They must also be designed to assist the nurse in explaining the ethical, moral, and value issues which impinge on the nursing practice and influence the impact the practice will have on the health care of society.

Emphasis on the substance of the objectives has been stressed at this point to focus on the need for validity of objectives. A perfectly worded objective that is completely out of the realm of reality is of little use to one seeking continued education experiences. The variety of sources that the program planner goes to for the focus of the behavioral objectives will enable the individual to avoid getting into a rut with programs. Too often, program planners tend to have the subject matter of programs arise from a limited vision of their work world so that programs become repetitive and boring and do little to expand the horizons of the practitioners.

TARGET POPULATION

Continuing education programs are designed for a very specific population—adult learners who are primarily engaged in the practice of nursing. Employment means a continuing involvement in the practice which influences the nurse's decision as to need for further education. The origin of the need from the work setting may be a positive factor in that it provides a source of motivation for the nurse's involvement in the program. However, it may also be an impediment to the nurse's decision making, for the experience may have fostered "tunnel vision" so that the greater parameters of nursing practice may not be recognized. Program planners are then challenged to develop behavioral objectives that help these nurses recognize their own need to expand their perspective of nursing.

Knowledge of the characteristics of the population group is as essential for writing behavioral objectives for continuing education programs as it is for any other type of educational program. Employment variables must be included in the development of a group's profile, for there is a close relationship between area of practice and attendance at continuing education programs. The profile of the target population is particularly significant in planning learning behavior outcomes, for the level of achievement designated must be compatible with the background of the population.

Recognition of adult learning principles is especially significant as program objectives are developed. The adult learner's need to be involved in the learning process requires that objectives reflect action and participation.

Too many programs are really "show and tell." Experts come before a group to show their wares and tell what they know. The learner can choose how much or how little involvement is desired. With no provision for active involvement in the process, the adult learner becomes tuned out and frustrated in the effort to relate the new learning to individual experiences. The interest in problem solving, the search for fulfillment of individually designated goals, and the ability to be self-directing are essential attributes of the adult learner which must be addressed in any continuing education program planning and must be reflected in the objectives stated for the program.

WRITING OF BEHAVIORAL OBJECTIVES

The format for writing behavioral objectives as described in Chapter 3 remains the same for the behavioral objectives prepared for continuing education programs. The particular nature of these programs, however, demands special considerations in determining the outcome as identified in the selection of the behavioral verb.

Selection of Action Verb

One of the first considerations in writing the behavioral objectives is the selection of the appropriate verb to connote the intended behavioral outcome. The list of verbs identified for each level of the three taxonomies that appear in Chapter 4 is most useful in designating the outcome. These verbs make our objectives more precise in meaning and facilitate communication between the program planner and the target population. Because of the characteristics of the audience and the goal of continuing education programs to assist the nurse in using new knowledge, the verbs identified in the first level of the cognitive and affective domains would be inappropriate. Listing or defining behaviors is primarily recall and requires no comprehension of the phenomena described. The following objective is appropriate for users of knowledge at the graduate nurse level.

The learner relates ethical theories to the decisions nurses make within the context of their practice.

The verb must also reflect a behavior that can be achieved within the limitations imposed by structure and time. Objectives that must be met outside the conference cannot be stated unless the program is a series extended over a period of time with practice planned for the intervening periods.

EXAMPLE: *The learner participates within the maternity nurse's professional role during the patient's delivery period.*

It is most probable that this behavior could not be met in a workshop of a day or two. However, the conceptual behavior could be achieved.

The learner describes the professional role of the maternity nurse during the patient's delivery period.

The development of a skill to a certain level of competency within a one- or two-day workshop is also questionable. This time frame provides for practice in the skill, but skill development demands more than most such workshops can provide. A behavior, then, might reflect a process inherent in the workshop rather than a direct outcome.

The application skill as expressed by such verbs as *use* and *apply* are more appropriate for longer workshops, where time allows for practice. Some formats that call for a one- or two-day session followed by assignments to be carried out in the work setting and then a meeting at a later date may have objectives that are behaviorally expressed as application relative to nursing practice. If the workshop provides practice sessions with the use of such skills as communication, problem solving, and decision making, the behaviors may be expressed as application outcomes.

The following objective is most appropriate for a skill in a one- or two-day continuing education program.

The learner practices techniques appropriate to the assessment of the adult's nervous system.

There are times when the behavioral objectives for a short-term workshop will be expressed in terms of the process behaviors rather than the outcome behaviors. Terms appropriate for such objectives are:

challenge	interact
communicate with	participate
contribute	practice
examine	question
explore	share ideas, concerns, etc.

NUMBER OF BEHAVIORAL OBJECTIVES

The number of behavioral objectives appropriate for a program depends on the intent of the program and its length. For most programs, the range of behavioral objectives is from four to six, a number which is most realistic for achievement, although even fewer objectives may be appropriate. At least one behavioral objective should be addressed to the relationship of the topic to nursing practice, for that legitimizes the program. The science theory is usually reflected in another behavior. Other objectives may relate to actual processes of the workshop activities such as *participates, explores, uses a problem-solving approach,* etc. Societal issues may also be indicated, and when psychomotor skills, interview skills, etc. are included, they need to be identified at the appropriate level of competency.

TESTING FOR CONTINUING
EDUCATION PROGRAMS

Should objectives written for continuing education programs be subject to testing as an evaluation method? Some programs do have protocols for testing which may include pre- and post-testing or written tests given to the attendees at the conclusion of the program. The response to this question is dependent on several factors: purpose of the program, the type of learning activities needed to attain the objectives, and the time frame within which the program is offered. Another major consideration relates to the attendees, most of whom are adults, and the recognized knowledge about how adults learned.

Previously, it was noted that for a one or two day program process rather than outcome objectives are recommended. This is an acknowledgement that in a limited time period the value of the program lies more in the learning achieved through experiencing than that which is obtained in synthesis. In many instances, when testing is instituted for these short-term programs, the questions are limited to the lower levels of the cognitive taxonomy, especially recall. Such a practice is inappropriate for individuals who are already practitioners in the field and adult learners.

Continuing education programs which extend over a longer period of time, where one has the opportunity to explore the meanings of new ideas and knowledge and perhaps practice in their use, are more amenable to testing, especially at the higher levels of the taxonomy. The objectives for such a program would be stated as outcome rather than the processes that occur in the program itself. Holzemer (1988) cautions about the limitations in the use of pre- and post-test as means of assessing learner outcomes. The question of internal validity needs to be raised with this approach for "there is no way to determine whether the observed change in scores is due to artifacts in the instrument, learning that occurred outside of the CE program, or any other variable" (p. 151). With these longer programs, a post-test could be used, especially if followed up by further data several months after the experience.

Although not all programs are suitable for testing learner outcomes, all programs can be evaluated in terms of the stated objectives. Holzemer (1988) refers to the most frequently used type of evaluation as "Happiness Index," which is useful in providing information about the program itself and the environmental factors, such as space, accommodations, and food. Such evaluation does not provide data on learning outcome, but is helpful for future planning. Several types of questions are helpful in enabling the participants to think about the knowledge component during the evaluation. These might be: How do you perceive using your experiences here within your practice? What learning during this program was new to you? What additional knowledge do you need before you feel you can use the learning from this program in your practice? Why would you feel that the knowledges explored in this program could not be used in your practice in the agency where you work?

These are only some ways at seeing where the participants are in relation to the knowledge component when the program is of short duration. It is true that such open-ended questions are not easy to review, but they could provide some valuable information to the planners and help to focus on the meaning of the experience. Some of these questions could be developed within a more structured format with option for the responders to add their own perceptions.

SUMMARY

The process of behavioral objective writing for continuing education programs represents many components, namely: the content to be addressed, the characteristics of the target population, the selection of action appropriate to the level of the learner and the time frame available, and the appropriateness of the objective to the nature of and setting of the continuing education offering. All of these components must be considered in preparing any set of objectives for a continuing education program.

Continuing education programs have special characteristics defined by their target population, which is composed of adult practitioners, and the limitations imposed by time and the scope of content restrictions. Their primary purpose is to facilitate the continued development of the practitioners and their practice. These characteristics demand that the program planner select appropriate behavioral objectives which are meaningful and achievable. Once the behavioral objectives are developed, they become a contract with the consumer and the continuing educator is accountable for developing a program congruent with the stated intent. All programs are to be evaluated, but testing is appropriate primarily for those extending over a sufficient period of time to enable learning to become internalized.

REFERENCES

Holzemer, W. (1988). Evaluation methods in continuing education. *Journal of Continuing Education in Nursing, 19*(4), 148–157.

Reilly, D. (1976). Preparation of objectives for continuing education programs. *Occupational Health Nursing, 24*(12), 30–33.

RECOMMENDED READINGS

Argyris, C., & Schön, D. (1974). *Theory in practice: Increasing professional effectiveness.* San Francisco: Jossey-Bass.

Bigge, M. (1982). *Learning theories for teachers* (4th ed.). New York: Harper & Row.

Bille, D. (1983). *Staff development: A systems view.* Thorofare, NJ: Charles Slack.

Daley, B. (1987). Goal-attainment scaling: A method of evaluation, Part one. *Journal of Continuing Education in Nursing, 18*(6), 200–202.

Daley, B. (1987). Applying goal-attainment scaling to nursing continuing education courses, Part two. *Journal of Continuing Education in Nursing, 18*(6), 203–208.

Dickinson, G., Holzemer, W., & Nichols, E. (1985). Evaluation of an arthritis continuing education program. *Journal of Continuing Education in Nursing, 16*(4), 127–131.

Hefferin, E. (1987). Trends in the evaluation of nursing inservice programs. *Journal of Nursing Staff Development, 3*(1), 28–40.

Kennedy, M. (1983). Designing and implementing successful continuing educational programs. *Journal of Continuing Education in Nursing, 16*(1), 16–20.

Kidd, J. (1976). *How adults learn.* New York: Associated Press.

Knox, A. (1977). *Adult development and learning.* San Francisco: Jossey-Bass.

Puetz, B., & Faye, L. (1981). *Continuing education for nurses: A complete guide for effective programs.* Rockville, MD: Aspen Systems.

Reilly, D. (1981). Why objectives? Relationship to occupational health nursing practice. *Occupational Health Nursing, 19*(6), 1–11.

Still, M. (1987). Continuing education for consensus on entry skills. *Journal of Professional Nursing, 3*(4), 214–217.

Wake, M. (1987). Effective instruction in continuing nursing education. *Journal of Continuing Education in Nursing, 18*(6), 188–192.

Yeaw, E. (1987). A theoretical model based on evaluation theories and application to continuing education programs in nursing. *Journal of Continuing Education in Nursing, 18*(40), 123–128.

7

Evaluation

Throughout the discussion of behavioral objectives, frequent reference was made to the relationship between objectives and evaluation. Behavioral objectives provide the *what* and suggest clues for the *how* of evaluation, unless they are expressed as specific behavioral objectives as in the behaviorism model. In this latter form, the specifics of the *how* are included in the behavioral objective.

In the vast amount of literature about educational evaluation, one concept that consistently appears is usually stated in the following manner: *evaluation is related to objectives* and is *delineated in terms of measurable student behavior*. Evaluation is a complex, multidimensional process, but the discussion in this book will be directed to that aspect of evaluation in an educational endeavor that is associated with behavioral objectives.

There are several misconceptions or patterns of thought about the concept of evaluation that must be explored here.

A review of the literature about evaluation, unless in reference to a specific type such as practice/clinical, suggests that the predominant emphasis within the topic relates to testing. Thus, the notions of testing and evaluation have become synonymous. This is unfortunate for tests are only one method of evaluation. The potential for a myriad of evaluation strategies is lost and all anxieties and concerns with testing become ascribed to evaluation. The whole premise behind open-ended objectives is the freedom of the teachers and learners to use evaluation in a more facilitative and dynamic

123

way. Unfortunately, the opportunities for creative approaches to evaluate are circumscribed usually by the limitations of the evaluators.

In addition, for many the relationship of testing and evaluation confirms that evaluation is a function of summarization of attainment of objectives, often allocating a quantitative value since most tests are ascribed a numerical value. Thus, students express negative feelings toward the experience of testing. Evaluation approaches, on the other hand, can be closely integrated as part of the learning experience, and, when challenging, can lead the learner into the excitement of discovery; discovery of self and discovery of new meanings in the phenomenon under study.

The perception of this close interrelationship between testing and evaluation ignores the significant role evaluation plays in the teaching process and its integration in learning. More will be said later about the critical role for formative evaluation which should occur whenever teacher and learner are engaged in the dynamic of learning. It is the learning process that is the focus of this evaluation, not the learning outcome.

Another misconception particularly relevant to evaluation is the lack of distinction between the terms *behavior*, *response*, and *behaviorism*, a natural science theory of learning. This distinction was discussed early, but bears reiteration here. The tendency to equate these two terms can be found in the professional literature. Diekelmann (1989) expressed this position, "The commitment to teaching as evaluation reflects behavioral education. Learning as a change in behavior and evaluation as evidence of it are the hallmarks of behavioral approaches" (p. 26).

When one learns new knowledge, skill, or values, one acts differently whether dealing with recall of facts, explanation of a process, or engaging in critical thinking or problem solving. A nursing student who has mastered skill in the use of problem solving for a clinical practice problem acts differently than before the skill was achieved when encountering a similar clinical problem. There has been a change in behavior and that is the emphasis of the learning outcome. Skill in use of problem solving for a clinical problem is the objective. The questions for the instructors are: What behaviors indicate that the skill has been attained, and what evaluation strategies can be used to ascertain the presence of these behaviors?

This example is not governed by behaviorism theory in which the learning process is mechanistic and all contingencies in the learning situation are stated in the objective including the evaluation strategy and criteria. Rather it denotes the competency to be attained and the context within which that behavior will be evaluated. The process by which the student learns the skill and the means by which it is evaluated are functions of the instructor's concept of the learning process.

The instructor's belief about evaluation and the energy and creativity brought to the process have a significant effect on the student's learning. Bigge (1982) reiterates this concept when he says, "The nature of the teacher's system for evaluation of student learning has a very great influence upon the quality of learning that actually develops" (p. 292). Some of the areas of influence identified by Bigge include a student's study habits, manner of interaction in class, number and quality of learnings, and the teaching–learning level upon which the student's learning efforts proceed.

ATTITUDES TOWARD EVALUATION

Evaluation is a judgmental process and, as such, it reflects the beliefs, values, and attitudes of participants. A critical determinant of the direction of evaluation is how the evaluator defines the term *evaluation*. As previously stated, *value* is part of the word formation, and since value is a personal concept, evaluation must be subjective.

Within the educational system of our society, evaluation has ordinarily been associated with grading performance and classifying students. More will be said later about the differences between these two processes. Since many associate evaluation with grading and classifying individuals and since our society uses these grades and/or classifications for many purposes, nurse teachers are asked to assume an awesome responsibility. Their judgment of a learner influences the student's job opportunities, choice of a career, acceptance and continuation in a program of studies, and even the student's social and personal identity within the matrix of society itself. As evaluators, faculty and other teachers in nursing are in a position to influence the destiny of learners with whom they are involved for their judgment is the one accepted by society.

One significant question must be answered by each nurse teacher, because the response determines the approach taken toward evaluation. Is evaluation a process for growth, or is it a means for control? The answer will come from the teacher's beliefs about the learner, the nature of the learner, and the nature of the teaching–learning process. The answer also will determine whether the teacher will ask the right questions, use the right evaluation method, and see the right behavior with respect to the learning experience.

Present use of evaluation in our society supports a negative connotation. As a result, we find that the behaviors accompanying evaluation reflect:

Anxiety instead of anticipation

Punishment instead of reward

Defeatism instead of encouragement

Compliance instead of self-determination

Safety instead of risk taking

Many nurse teachers support the premise that a primary goal in living is the individual's ability to know the self and to develop progressively to fulfill his or her potential. Evaluation is a major process in helping the individual to achieve self-actualization, yet as customarily used, evaluation has not consistently helped others to realize this goal. Instead, self-knowledge may be considered so frightening that a defensive approach to evaluation becomes a common pattern of behavior.

No doubt evaluation carries a strong power component and use of this power is circumscribed by the evaluator's perception of the process. Some individuals have a consistent need to control others, thus evaluation can be a potent weapon. Unfortunately, all helping professions appear to attract these "controllers of man," for these professions concern themselves with individuals or groups who are more or less dependent. Controllers base their evaluation on rules, regulations, and procedures, tending to manipulate the learner in order to fit behavior into the accepted code. Learners are then forced to direct their energies toward surviving in the system, rather than toward experiences that would contribute to growth and development.

The power component, however, also is used by evaluators who are facilitators and who perceive evaluation as related to the learner's growth. These individuals accept the concept of mastery of learning, and, by using evaluation as a diagnostic process, develop teaching strategies that stimulate the learners to search for self-knowledge and to develop their potential. Rules, regulations, and procedures are not ends in themselves but means to ends that best serve the learner and other persons in a particular setting. Here, facilitators promote student involvement in the evaluation of the learning process and learning outcome.

The power potential in evaluation also affects evaluators who perceive the process in terms of themselves rather than as a growth process for the student. The student's success or failure is equated with the teacher's success or failure. If students succeed, it often goes unnoticed, but if a student fails, the teacher responds as though the failure were a personal one. Guilt, self-recrimination, and depression are often the result.

In this situation, the teacher assumes his or her role is omnipotent. A belief in mastery of learning approach does not mean complete success for all students, because many variables associated with learning, including motivation and persistence, are ostensibly controlled by the learner. Failure requires an honest appraisal of all factors impinging on the teaching–learning process in order to establish a diagnosis and develop a suggested prescription for treatment. The diagnosis may indeed suggest faculty failure, or student failure, or even failure resulting from extraneous sources beyond the control of student or teacher.

CONCEPT OF THE PROCESS

Evaluation was defined previously as a process concerned with determining the quality of a substance, action, or event. In the context of education, evaluation refers to a process or combination of processes whereby nurse teachers judge student accomplishments relative to specific behavioral objectives.

Bloom, Hastings, and Madaus (1971) express the following views about evaluation that connote the major purposes:

1. *Evaluation as a method of acquiring and processing the evidence needed to improve student learning and teaching.*

2. *Evaluation as including a great variety of evidence beyond the usual final paper and pencil examination.*

3. *Evaluation as an aid in clarifying the significant goals and objectives of education and as a process of determining the extent to which students are developing in these desired ways.*

4. *Evaluation as a system of quality control in which it may be determined at each step in the learning process whether the process is effective or not, and if not, what changes must be made to insure its effectiveness before it is too late.*

5. *Evaluation as a tool in educational practice for ascertaining whether or not alternative procedures are equally effective in achieving a set of educational ends* (p. 8).

These views depict a vibrant, dynamic, continuous, open-ended process closely interwoven with the teaching–learning process. They are in sharp contrast to the all-too-frequently expressed view of evaluation as synonymous with grading or ranking students. The rationale for evaluation relates to assessment for growth: growth of the learner, growth of the teacher, growth of the teaching–learning process, and ultimately growth of the program and the institution offering the program.

Evaluation is not an end in itself, it is a means to an end. The process can enhance the students' personal development and learning or destroy the incentive to learn and distort personality development. Teachers should use evaluation wisely, consistent with developmental concepts of teaching–learning.

Two terms regarding evaluation are in current use today—*summative* evaluation and *formative* evaluation. Summative evaluation occurs at the end of a program, course, or unit, and refers to the extent to which the learner has realized all of specified behavioral objectives. Formative evaluation occurs throughout the program, course, and unit, and refers to the learner's progress toward realizing behavioral objectives. It states what is and what can be.

Summative evaluation is the more common practice in many programs; it is used to determine grades, certify students, and sometimes to judge the teacher's effectiveness. Tests or papers at midterm or final periods are the usual procedures. In this type of evaluation, there is a concept of finality, stating what is rather than what is and what can be.

The concept of formative evaluation is generally accepted in principle by many teachers, but a gap exists between expressed belief and action. This type of evaluation operates throughout the learning process and is concerned with the learner's progress during the learning period, not at the end of it. Formative evaluation relies on feedback to guide the learner and the teacher to aspects of learning that need critical attention as the learner moves toward mastery of the behavior.

Williams (1985), in his excellent article, "Effective Teaching: Gauging Learning While Teaching," addresses the issue of formative evaluation in the discussion of warning signs that students are not understanding the material being presented. He comments on experiences that faculty have when students perform poorly on tests when the content, although somewhat difficult, seemed to be understood by the students as evidenced by students' behavior. The tendency of faculty to rely on how students appear (visual feedback) can be misleading and not a true measure of their level of understanding. Analysis of research suggests that verbal cues are more indicative of understanding for they relate to the cognitive processing level of the students. Williams's conclusion is that, "observing many student verbal behaviors indicating a deeper level of processing (accompanied by selected visual cues like alertness, eye contact, attention posture, active note-taking) should indicate that a desirable level of student understanding is being achieved" (pp. 335–336). In a class situation, although the quality of verbal cues is important, the teacher must also note the number of students participating through offering verbal cues and assure that the climate of the classroom is supportive of students' efforts to deal with new and challenging ideas. Williams has presented suggestions for use of formative evaluation with large classes, particularly lecture periods. This is more difficult than in small group classes and individual learning situations. Formative evaluation is no less important with the larger classes and behavior of students is a critical dimension for evaluation.

Varieties of evaluation procedures may be used. These include written tests, problem situations, observation of behaviors in practice or group situations, conferences, and videotaping. The important point is that these procedures are not designed for grading a student but to assess progress, to diagnose learning needs so that remedial measures can be instituted promptly, and to pace the student's learning to individual needs and abilities. At the present time, formative evaluation is used sporadically in nursing programs and is usually directed to the poor student. A commitment to evaluation as an integral part of the teaching–learning process requires that a systematic approach to formative evaluation be developed and that summative evaluation be used periodically.

PSYCHOSOCIAL CLIMATE OF EVALUATION

Evaluation is presented as a positive process whose primary purpose is to assess growth. But, it was previously noted that many individuals involved in education do not view evaluation in this light. Practice, then, often has not been congruent with the belief that evaluation is a process directed toward development. How might participants in the teaching–learning process enjoy a positive experience in evaluation?

The critical variable in evaluation is the psychosocial climate prevailing during the process. The climate includes beliefs, values, feeling tones, and attitudes regarding evaluation of participants and the nature of the relationships existing among them. Rogers (1983) refers to the attitudinal qualities of interpersonal relationships between facilitator and learner when he states:

> *First of all is a transparent realness in the facilitator, a willingness to be a person, to be and live the feelings and thoughts of the moment. When this realness includes a prizing, a caring, a trust, and respect for the learner, the climate for learning is enhanced. When it includes a sensitive and accurate empathic listening, then, indeed, a freeing climate stimulative of self initiated learning and growth exists. The student is TRUSTED to develop* (p. 133).

Maintaining the climate proposed by Rogers depends on the teacher's actions in the situation, for it is through actions that the student is able to assess the teacher's intent. One action that provides this facilitative environment for the evaluation experience is the use of behavioral objectives.

Behavioral objectives communicate to the learner the behaviors expected to be developed and on which evaluation is to be based. If, in evaluating the student, the teacher adheres to the Pntentof the behavior, the student is free to learn and does not need to expend energy on outsmarting the instructor in preparation for evaluation. Behavioral objectives discipline the teacher to evaluate the behavior indicated in the contract with the student. Thus, the teacher cannot focus on extraneous behaviors in an assessment, and teacher hang ups or biases are excluded. How often have evaluations of the nurse's behavior in a clinical practice setting paid minimal heed to competency in clinical practice but included numerous comments relative to length of hair, condition of uniform, or posture. Evaluations of this latter type do much to undermine the climate of trust, and force the learner into playing games in an effort to survive. The survival need, and not the learning need, becomes the motivating force.

The climate described by Rogers predicates an environment in which learning includes opportunity for intelligent risk taking. A developmental learning experience must provide students with opportunities to explore ideas and methods. A climate that values safety discourages the inquiring student, for the risks at evaluation time are too great. Rewards may be based on the results of the endeavor rather than on the process involved in the endeavor. Thus, the creative learner who dares to move from the tried path often is evaluated by a standard that frequently incorporates the utilitarian concept, "Is it workable?"

In too many instances, nurse teachers are uncomfortable with intelligent risk taking, and safety is the predominating criterion used in providing student learning experience. Safety as referred to in this instance is unrelated to the reality of the situation and is usually a reflection of the teacher's insecurity and reliance on rules and past patterns of action. Intelligent risk taking means the decision to take a novel action after the consequences of such an action have been considered. In most learning endeavors there is room for error, and, indeed, learning from mistakes is a creditable concept. Nursing programs, however, seek perfection in practice and allow little margin for error in the learning situation. Fear of error again restrains the learner from developing potential, for a record of errors becomes the content of many evaluations.

Prather (1970) provides some insight into the role of mistakes in an individual's development.

> *Perfection is slow death. If everything*
> *were to turn out just like I would want it*
> *to, just like I would plan for it to, then I* .
> *would never experience anything new; my life*
> *would be an endless repetition of stale*

successes. When I make a mistake I experience
something unexpected.

    I sometimes react to making a mistake as
if I have betrayed myself. My fear of making
a mistake seems to be based on the hidden
assumption that I am potentially perfect and
that if I can just be very careful, I will
not fall from heaven. But a "mistake" is a
declaration of the way I AM, a jolt to the
way I intend, a reminder I am not dealing with
facts. When I have listened to my mistakes,
I have grown.

Can students listen to their own mistakes? Are nurse teachers secure enough to permit students to listen to their mistakes? Formative evaluation should support the student's listening and help in finding new directions. A formative evaluation based on a concept of perfection is not one that supports the student in the search for self-knowledge and in developing potential. A climate in which mistakes are permitted to occur and provision is made for intelligent risk taking as part of the learning process must be characterized by respect, trust, realness, and caring about the participants. It is under these conditions that evaluation can be accepted as a component of the teaching–learning process.

DIFFERENCES BETWEEN THE GRADING AND THE EVALUATION PROCESSES

Reference has been made to the fact that evaluation often is equated with grading. Frequently, when various types of evaluation procedures are discussed, the question is raised: How does one arrive at a grade from each procedure? Yet the concept of formative evaluation is not based on the premise of grading, but rather concerns itself with assessment for learner's guidance. Thus, all evaluation cannot be translated into grades.

    Evaluation and grading are two separate processes. Whereas evaluation has been described as the process by which teachers make judgments about student achievement of designated behavioral objectives, grading is the process by which teachers assign symbols that represent the student's level of academic achievement. Grading has a quantitative dimension; evaluation has a qualitative dimension. The grading process then follows the evaluation process. Evaluation can occur without grading; grading should not occur without evaluation.

Grading is generally associated with summative evaluation, and translation of results of the evaluation is the most significant phase in the grading process. Unless the grade conveys sufficient information when it is interpreted, it has little value. The data base for any grade consists of whatever kinds of evidence a particular faculty member determines are indicators of student achievement as defined by that teacher. These components are then weighted and combined into a single scale by some formula developed by the faculty member. A symbol is then designated according to the student's placement on the scale. In reference to grades, Warren (1971) says:

> Grades may therefore be accurate in reflecting performance on some undefined dimension of academic achievement. But their fidelity is poor in that they transmit only a small part of the information in the evaluations that led to the grade, while leaving the information they do transmit difficult to interpret (p. 2).

Reilly and Oermann (1985) identify several variables which influence the meaning behind grades, and thus raise questions about grades themselves: Do they truly represent the value of the evaluation data? Reilly and Oermann indicate reasons why standardization of grades does not exist.

1. *The person who grades has elements in own life space and a value system by which the meaning of grades is determined.*

2. *Inconsistency in quality and quantity of the evaluation data base exists among persons assigning grades. Some may use only one measure (i.e., paper or test) while others use a multiple of evaluation data sources.*

3. *Consistency with which the data base truly reflects the stated objectives may not be maintained.*

4. *Differing bases for standards in determining grades exist whereby some grades are based on process, some on outcome and some are based on both.*

5. *Inconsistency in the computation methods among graders exists in determining how grades are reached. Some use a norm referenced approach such as the normal curve while others use a criterion-referenced approach such as mastery of learning.*

6. *The weighing of different data sources follow different procedures among graders.*

The issues relative to grading and its place in higher education are beyond the limits of this book. The discussion presented here is meant to clarify the difference between the evaluation and the grading processes, the former as a judgment of quality and the latter as a quantitative measurement. It is important for faculty to realize that the grade is ordinarily not a reliable and valid basis for evaluating a student's performance unless accompanied by a teacher's descriptive evaluation of the student's achievement.

NEED FOR A VARIETY OF EVALUATION STRATEGIES

It has been pointed out that evaluation is an integral part of the teaching-learning process and that it contributes to the learner's development. Because it is interwoven in the student's total educational experiences, a variety of approaches must be used. No one evaluation strategy is sufficient for all learners in all situations.

The following are five significant reasons for providing diversity in evaluation strategies.

1. *Complexity of human behavior.* Human behavior is a phenomenon representing the motivations, values, needs, experiences, and perceptions of an individual at any point in time. It is variable, changeable, open-ended, and responsive to stimuli from both the internal and external environment. Any process for appraising behavior must reflect recognition of its multidimensional character and include suitable methods that consider its complexity.

2. *Individual differences in response to learning.* Each individual's response to learning reflects his or her abilities, interests, experiences, values, needs, beliefs, motivations, and perceptions. The learner has developed an individual style of learning and has become selective in the types of stimuli responded to in a learning situation. In any learning experience, no two individuals are alike in all dimensions. Evaluation processes, then, must provide for individual responses to any learning situation.

3. *Suitability of specific evaluation approaches to specific types of learning behaviors.* Learning behaviors have been classified within three domains: cognitive, affective, and psychomotor. Each of these domains calls on different abilities in the learner and requires different strategies for determining its behavioral attainment. As an example, an observation evaluation strategy is more appropriate for

identifying a psychomotor competency than is a response on written paper.

4. *Motivational factor of evaluation.* Evaluation, especially formative evaluation, is designed to help the learner improve performance while still in the process of learning the behavior designated by the behavioral objective. It relies on feedback to help both the teacher and the learner diagnose learning needs and intervene with appropriate teaching strategies. Evaluation that uses feedback and involves the learner in the appraisal is a significant factor in helping the learner to become self-motivating. Again, the use of various methods (especially in terms of the focus of the evaluation and the individuality of the student) can be helpful in the student's perception of the evaluation process as a means for self growth.

5. *Creative dimension to the evaluation process.* Like other teaching and learning strategies, evaluation strategies are most open to the teacher's and learner's creativity. An open-ended system of teaching promotes the acceptance of novelty in evaluation approaches to behavioral objectives, which often add vitality to the process. In too many instances, evaluation procedures are embedded in the "cement" of the educational program and become boring to students and teachers. In creating new evaluation methods or protocols, risk taking plays an integral part. Sharing in a new venture can be a stimulating experience to both students and teachers, especially if all are involved in assessing the evaluation strategy itself. Evaluation practices need not be in a rut; they can be creative, and therefore limited only by the extent of the imagination of participants and by their perseverance in pursuing the development, implementation, and assessment of practices.

The challenge then rests with the teacher who must develop and use evaluation strategies that are meaningful, relevant, and stimulating to the learner.

SUMMARY

Evaluation is the process or combination of processes whereby a teacher judges a student's accomplishment relative to specified behavioral objectives. The psychosocial climate in which this process occurs influences the effectiveness of the process. An environment characterized by respect, trust, empathy, caring, and risk taking facilitates the evaluation process as an integral part of the teaching–learning process geared toward student growth and development. An environment created by individuals who need to control others fosters the use of evaluation as a force of control and directs student energy into game playing for survival rather than into learning pursuits.

Two types of evaluation are in current use. Formative evaluation occurs throughout the program, course, or unit, and through feedback enables teacher and student to diagnose learning needs, to provide appropriate remedial strategies, and to pace the student's learning according to his needs and abilities. Summative evaluation occurs at the end of the program, course, or unit and is concerned with the extent to which the learner has mastered all designated behavioral objectives. It is usually associated with grading but is not synonymous with it. Summative evaluation relates to the judgment a teacher makes about student achievement, whereas grading is the process by which the teacher assigns symbols that represent specific levels of student achievement.

Since evaluation is inherent in an effective teaching–learning process, varieties of strategies are indicated. Reasons for this variety are:

1. Complexity of human behavior.
2. Individual differences in learning.
3. Suitability of specific evaluation approaches to specific types of learning.
4. Motivational factor in evaluation.
5. The creative dimension to the evaluation process.

REFERENCES

Bigge, M. (1982). *Learning theories for teaching* (4th ed.). New York: Harper & Row.

Bloom, B., Hastings, J., & Madaus, G. (1971). *Handbook on formative and summative evaluation of student learning.* New York: McGraw-Hill.

Diekelmann, N. (1989). The nursing curriculum: Lived experiences of students. In National League for Nursing. *Curriculum revolution: Reconceptualizing nursing education* (pp. 25–42). New York: National League for Nursing.

Prather, H. (1970). *Notes to myself.* Utah: Real People Press.

Reilly, D., & Oermann, M. (1985). *The clinical field: Its use in nursing education.* Norwalk, CT: Appleton-Century-Crofts.

Rogers, C. (1983). *Freedom to learn in the 80's.* Columbus, OH: Charles Merrill.

Warren, J. (1971). *College grading practices: An overview.* Washington, DC: ERIC Clearing House on Education.

Williams, W. C. (1985). Effective teaching: Gauging learning while teaching. *Journal of Higher Education, 56*(3), 320–327.

RECOMMENDED READINGS

Anderson, S., Scarvia, B., & Ball, S. (1978). *The profession and practice of program evaluation.* San Francisco: Jossey-Bass.

Beyer, F. (1983). Setting passing scores. *Nursing & Health Care, 4,* 518–522.

Dressel, P. (1980). Models for evaluating individual achievement. *Journal of Higher Education, 51,* 194–205.

Huckaby, L. (1979). Cognitive-affective consequences of grading vs non-grading of formative evaluations. *Nursing Research, 28,* 175–178.

James, M. (1987). Student perception of end of course evaluations. *Journal of Higher Education, 58,* 704–716.

Kegan, D. (1977). Using Bloom taxonomy for curriculum planning and evaluation in non-traditional settings. *Journal of Higher Education, 48,* 63–70.

Kolb, S., & Shugart, E. (1984). Evaluation: Is simulation the answer? *Journal of Nursing Education, 23,* 84–86.

Litwack, L., Linc, L., & Bower, D. (1985). *Evaluation in nursing: Principles and practice.* New York: National League for Nursing.

Milton, O., Pollio, H., & Eison, J. (1986). *Making sense of college grades.* San Francisco: Jossey-Bass.

Reilly, D. (1978). *Teaching and evaluating the affective domain.* Thorofare, NJ: Slack.

Rosen, M. (1983). Forecasting summative evaluation from formative evaluation: A double cross-validation study. *Psychological Reports, 49*(3), 843–848.

Schneider, H. (1979). *Evaluation of nursing competence.* Boston: Little Brown & Co.

8

Methods of Evaluating Attainment of Behavioral Objectives

Behavioral objectives are the substance of evaluation in educational programs. They specify the behavior to be evaluated and the content to which the behavior is related. The point is that there must be a direct connection between the behavioral objective and the evaluation procedure.

The evaluation procedure must be addressed to *what* of the behavioral objective. One of the first steps in assuring this relationship is to select an evaluation method that provides data relative to the student's achievement of the designated behavior. The evaluation method should be appropriate to a particular situation.

A second step, however, is to determine whether the evaluation procedure really tests the behavior under examination. The method of evaluation may indeed be appropriate for a particular behavior, but the task implied in the method may be unrelated to the behavior. A written essay question on a test may be selected as the methodology for evaluating the nursing student's competency in explaining a concept of the nursing process. But if the task implied in the written question calls on the student to list the steps in the process, the behavior of *explaining* is not being evaluated.

This chapter is concerned with the relationship between the *what* and *how* of evaluation. Various methods of evaluation suitable to nursing programs are discussed and illustrated in relation to specific behavioral objectives. In the following examples, the learner in the objectives is the nursing student and only the behavior will be stated. The nursing student refers to any learner in nursing, i.e., a student in a school of nursing, or a practitioner in a staff development program or a program of continuing education. The coding before each behavior refers to the taxonomies discussed in Chapter 4.

PAPER-AND-PENCIL TEST ITEMS

Alternate Response

Test items in this classification ask the student to match one meaning of a fact, idea, concept, or definition with the one presented. The student is asked to accept or reject the statement given. Forms of alternate response generally used are: true-false, accept-not accept, agree-disagree.

This form of test item is used most often in relation to the recall level of cognition. It is also effective in ascertaining beliefs and attitudes, the awareness or responding level of the affective domain. When students are directed to provide a rationale, the comprehension level of cognition is being evaluated, and the objective should be stated accordingly.

GENERAL PRINCIPLES OF CONSTRUCTION

The following are principles of construction:

1. The directions for answering the questions must be exact.
2. The truth or falsity should be expressed between subject and verb, never by a phrase tacked on at the end or by inserting an incidental phrase in the question.
3. Statements should be true or false without qualification.
4. The statement itself should be confined to one idea.
5. Specific determiners such as always, never, usually and generally should be avoided.
6. Long involved statements with many qualifying phrases should be avoided.
7. Negatively worded statement should be avoided.

8. There should be approximately the same number of false and true items.

9. A double space between items provides for easier reading.

10. Modifications can help to eliminate guessing. Suggestions include:

    a. explanation of false statement

    b. statement of reason for choice

    c. correction and/or revision of incorrect statement

Directions: For each of the following statements, circle "T" if the statement is true and "F" if the statement is false.

ILLUSTRATIONS

BEHAVIORAL OBJECTIVES	TEST ITEM
C1.25 Identifies primary sources of data collection for assessment of patient needs.	T.F. Consultation and patient interview are two primary sources of data collection relative to patient needs.
C1.32 Identifies the relationship between a pathological state and the signs and symptoms exhibited.	T.F. A decrease in breath sounds occurs in a condition such as atelectasis.
C1.11 Defines terminology referrent to diseases of the heart.	T.F. Endocarditis is an inflammation of the heart muscle.

(If evaluation is to be addressed to the cognitive level of comprehension, the following statement is added to the instructions: In the space below each statement, cite the rationale for your choice.)

C2.2 Differentiates between fact and stereotype about elderly people.	T.F. Old people are senile, ill, and nonproductive.
C2.2 Explains the relationship between oxygen concentration and physiological response.	T.F. Oxygen therapy in severe emphysema may result in apnea.

(If evaluation is to be addressed to the affective domain, the terms agree-disagree are used. The instructions then ask to circle the "A" or "D" instead of the "T" or "F".)

A1.1 Is aware that each individual has the right to quality nursing care.	A.D. The quality of nursing care needed for the substance abuser is different from that required by a college professor who is not a substance abuser.

BEHAVIORAL OBJECTIVES	TEST ITEM
A1.2 Acknowledges rights of patients.	A.D. Patients have the right to make decisions related to their plan of care.

Alternate response items are useful in testing a large area of content within a short period. They are easy to score unless an explanation is requested. They are useful in testing attitudes, misconceptions, and beliefs. In questions such as the ones listed above for the affective domain, responses should not be translated into grades. These kinds of questions are particularly good as part of the system of formative evaluation. Alternate response questions are subject to responses in which there is a large element of guessing unless the question requires justification for the response selected.

Multiple Recognition Questions

This format for questions provides students with several alternatives from which to choose the correct response. It is useful for the first three levels of the cognitive domain (knowledge, comprehension, and application) as well as for the first three levels in the affective domain (receiving, responding, and valuing). This format can be used in conjunction with maps, diagrams, and charts.

There are two forms for this type of question.

1. Multiple choice: one answer is selected from a number of plausible ones. It may be the one *correct* answer, the best of several *correct* answers, or the one *incorrect* answer.

2. Multiple response: several correct responses are possible, and the selection is based on the best combination of responses.

GENERAL PRINCIPLES OF CONSTRUCTION

The following are principles of construction:

1. The structure includes a statement (stem) and a list of responses (alternatives or distractors)
2. Forms of statement
    a. Incomplete sentence relying on the alternative to complete it
    b. Complete statement
    c. Question

3. Forms of distractors

 a. Single word

 b. Phrase

 c. Complete sentence

4. Principles regarding the statement (stem)

 a. The statement must include the nature of the response: Which of the following *responses, functions, etc.* (do not just say which of the following)

 b. If only one response is desired—state which *one* of the following (functions).

 c. If the statement is to be completed by the response, do not place a period at the end of the statement. The period is placed after each response.

 d. Do not end an incomplete statement with *a* or *an* as this may give a clue to the correct response (*an* indicates a distractor beginning with a vowel).

 e. If statement asks for a response that does not apply—underline the word *not* or *except* in the stem.

 f. Each question should be independent of other items to avoid presenting data in one question that helps answer another.

5. Principles regarding the *response* (correct answer and distractors)

 a. In any one question the response format must be consistent (i.e., all phrases, all one word, all complete sentences) to avoid giving clues as to the correct or incorrect response.

 b. If the response completes a statement, the first work of the response is in lower case and a period is at the conclusion of the response.

 c. If the response completes a statement, all responses must complete the statement grammatically.

 d. At least four responses should be included in any question.

 e. All responses should be logical and relevant to the statement.

 f. The length of the responses should be similar.

 g. Responses also should be similar in complexity and detail to avoid providing clues as to the correct or incorrect response.

 h. Responses that are obviously wrong or inappropriate weaken the questions; distractors should be plausible.

 i. No response should give a clue to the answer.

 j. All responses should be placed at the end of the stem.

k. Responses containing numerical values should be listed sequentially, and values should not overlap.

SPECIAL CONSIDERATIONS: MULTIPLE RESPONSE

1. Responses are generally identified as a letter.
2. The best combination of responses are identified by number. Instructions ask the student to circle the appropriate *number* preceding the best combination of responses.
3. There should be four or five combinations of responses.
4. In the combination, it is important that there be reasonable equity in selecting responses. Predominance in use of one letter or limited use of a letter provides clues to the correct response.
5. It is advisable to indent the alternatives and to line up the combination of responses with the statement.
6. The combination of responses should be listed sequentially, i.e., in a logical order.

BEHAVIORAL OBJECTIVES

Multiple Choice
C2.2 Distinguishes abnormal from normal body change in the aging process.

C1.22 Names the steps of the nursing process.

TEST ITEM

Instruction: Circle the letter preceding the process that correctly completes the following statement.

The body change which is *not* a usual characteristic of aging is
A. decrease in metabolism
B. loss in weight
C. loss of skin turgor
D. decrease in sensory function
E. frequency in urination

Instruction: Circle the letter preceding the correct sequence of steps in the nursing process.

The sequence of steps in the nursing process includes
A. evaluation, planning, assessment, intervention

BEHAVIORAL OBJECTIVES

TEST ITEM

B. intervention, planning, evaluation, assessment

C. assessment, planning, intervention, evaluation

D. assessment, intervention, planning, evaluation

A3.1 Responds supportively to parents' expressed concern about their child's care.

Instruction: Circle the letter preceding the best response to the parents' expressed concern.

Mary, a two-year-old, is receiving I.V. therapy and is restrained. Her father says to you, "I know she needs fluids, but I hate to see her tied up like this." Your best response is:

A. "She is restrained for her own good so she won't pull out the needle."

B. "We restrain all the children receiving I.V.s."

C. It is hard to see Mary restrained; the restraint is used so she will not dislodge the I.V. accidentally."

D. "We don't want her to pull out the I.V."

C1.21 Identifies physiological actions of exercise of joints.

Instruction: Circle the number preceding the best selection of responses.

Which of the following physiological actions occur with exercise of the knee?

A. Blood circulation is increased

B. Muscle tone is improved

C. Sensation in joints is lessened

D. Contractures are prevented

E. Mobility of joints is improved

   1. A, B, C

   2. A, B, D, E

   3. A, C, D

   4. B, C

   5. B, D, E

BEHAVIORAL OBJECTIVES

Multiple Response
C2.2   Detects clues in communication that connote a cultural interpretation of the time and/or space dimension.

TEST ITEM

Instruction: Circle the number preceding the best combination of responses.

Which of the following statements contain clues indicative of cultural interpretation of time and/or space?

A. "Yes, I will be available for an hour."
B. "Since the party starts at 6:30, I will invite him for 6:00."
C. "Stay away. Don't touch me."
D. "Anyone who has to get that close to speak to someone has something wrong."
   1. A, B, C
   2. A, B, D
   3. A, C, D
   4. B, C, D
   5. A, B, C, D

A3.1   Supports individuals in expressing grief.

Instruction: Circle the number preceding the best combination of responses.

Since Ms. D was notified that there is now lung involvement from metastases of her breast cancer, she has become withdrawn and speaks only when spoken to. Which of the following goals would you set for your nursing intervention?

A. Respect Ms. D's right to be silent
B. Protect Ms. D from becoming emotionally upset
C. Encourage Ms. D to talk about her feelings regarding her illness
D. Keep Ms. D from morbidly dwelling on her illness

BEHAVIORAL OBJECTIVES

TEST ITEM

E. Keep staff informed as to Ms. D's method of handling her illness
1. A, B, C, E
2. A, B, D
3. A, C, D, E
4. A, C, E
5. B, C, D

Multiple recognition questions like alternate choice questions are useful in testing large areas of content. This form is used widely in our educational system, both for tests on course material and for standardized tests used nationally and internationally. They are used less frequently in other countries and thus international students applying for admission to schools in the United States may be handicapped when they are used. Also, because the distractors are so specific, this question format is particularly susceptible to cultural bias.

Some educators see limitations in their use, particularly with creative students who are distracted by the ambiguity and simplification of the distractors. These students often see greater implications in the question than suggested by the choice of distractors. A further concern with this format relates to the technique used by some students in responding; they become test-wise. Response is then less an indication of the knowledge of the student than it reflects skill in taking these kinds of tests.

Completion Questions

These questions require students to complete a statement by inserting the missing words or phrases. The format may be sentences or paragraphs. This format is used primarily for the recall level of cognition with reference to definitions, specific terms, and facts.

GENERAL PRINCIPLES OF CONSTRUCTION

1. Blanks used at the end of a sentence simplify scoring.
2. Too many blanks in a statement should be avoided as the question could become puzzling.
3. All blanks should be standard length.

4. Key words are the ones to be omitted.

5. The use of *a* or *an* immediately preceding a blank should be avoided.

6. Only one answer should be possible for each blank.

BEHAVIORAL OBJECTIVES	TEST ITEM
	Instruction: Complete the blanks.
C1.12 Names community resources designed to meet the needs of mentally retarded children and their families.	Two community resources available to the parents of mentally retarded children are _____ and _____.
C1.11 Identifies a concept of integrity.	According to Erikson, the ability to look back on one's life with satisfaction is indicative of the achievement of _____.
C1.24 Identifies characteristics of sounds elicited when using auscultation technique.	The clear, long, low-pitched sound elicited over the normal lung is called _____.

Completion questions are useful in testing facts, but care must be taken that the blanks do not lead to ambiguity or to confusion so that the student is prevented from getting the sense of the statement. Some educators feel that this type of question fosters rote memorization in the learning process.

Matching Questions

Like other forms of question discussed so far, this is an approach that provides for proficiency in terms of covering the content area of study. In this approach, the student is asked to relate facts, ideas, principles, or terms in one column to a statement or term in another column. Its primary use is at the recall level of the cognitive domain.

GENERAL PRINCIPLES OF CONSTRUCTION

1. Terms used should be stated clearly.

2. More choices should be listed in the right-hand column than items to be identified in the left-hand column. This eliminates the possibility of making choices by a process of elimination.

3. The terminology in the left-hand column should not give clues to the expected response in the right-hand column.

4. If each term in the right-hand column can be used more than once, this information should be included in the instructions.

5. The instructions should indicate the basis for matching.

6. The response list should be homogeneous in format.

ILLUSTRATIONS

BEHAVIORAL OBJECTIVE	TEST ITEM
C1.2 Defines the terms of techniques used in a physical examination.	*Instruction:* On the line to the left of each term in Column A, write the letter of the statement in Column B that matches the term.

Column A	Column B
_____ 1. Percussion	a. Use of the sense of touch to feel or press upon parts of the body.
_____ 2. Inspection	b. The striking of an area of the body with fingers or instruments and listening to sounds produced.
_____ 3. Palpation	c. Use of the sense of hearing to interpret sounds produced within the body.
_____ 4. Auscultation	d. Visual examination for detection of features or qualities perceptible to the eye.
	e. The act of perceiving what is detected by the senses.

This format is a useful method of testing recall. It requires attention to details in construction so that the match between the two columns is unambiguous but not obvious.

Essay Question

The essay question, particularly beyond the knowledge level of the cognitive domain, not only tests the student's information about the subject matter but also the student's ability to communicate ideas in a logical and coherent manner. It is used for all levels of the cognitive domain taxonomy, with the task called for in the question being the critical determinant of the level of cognition sought. The tasks signified for each level are stated similarly to the following.

Knowledge	How many, when, where, what name, list, define
Comprehension	Give illustrations, describe, explain, predict
Application	Give underlying principles, generalize, relate
Analysis	Analyze a problem, analyze data, compare, contrast, deduce
Synthesis	Formulate a new plan, design an approach, or write a perspective of an issue using relevant theories or concepts
Evaluation	Examine conclusions, judge accuracy, validity, reliability

The essay question, especially an open-ended one, is also useful in assessing development in the affective domain, especially at valuing or conceptualization levels. If an opinion is called for, the essay question is used only for formative evaluation, and the results cannot be graded. If, however, the cognitive base of the learner's opinion is requested, one may use the essay question in summative evaluation and translate the results into a grade. The opinion offered cannot be graded, but the logic of the rationale can be.

GENERAL PRINCIPLES OF CONSTRUCTION

1. The question should be constructed carefully so that the nature of the task is clearly stated. (The word discuss, used without a modifying phrase for direction, should be avoided, for it is too general a concept and does not give sufficient guidelines to the learner.)

2. The question should be constructed carefully so that exact limits of areas are clearly defined e.g., a concept such as "care of the cardiac patient" is complicated and multidimensional. The student needs to know the focus of deliberations intended for the question, such as: psychosocial, pathophysiological, or economic dimensions. More

than one dimension can be included in the question as long as the student knows the boundaries.

3. The desired outcome of the area tested should be set up as a basis for grading.

4. The student must know the basis of evaluation, especially when grading is to follow the evaluation. The basis might include:

   a. Evidence of meeting intended behaviors

   b. Evidence of the ability to select, organize, and present material in a coherent manner

5. When grading essay questions, critique one question for all students before advancing to the next question.

Questions arise as to the appropriateness of evaluating grammar and spelling. If the essay question is a part of the in-class examination, the grammar and spelling should be evaluated but not graded, unless inaccuracies interfere with a coherent presentation. In an out-of-class examination, however, where the student has access to references, spelling and grammar should be considered legitimate competencies in communicating ideas.

ILLUSTRATIONS OF TYPES OF ESSAY QUESTIONS

BEHAVIORAL OBJECTIVES	TEST ITEM
Knowledge Level	
C1.12 Recalls factors that influence a person's ability to adapt.	List five factors that have an influence on an individual's capacity to adapt.
C1.23 Names, in order, the stages of the grief process.	List, in order, the stages of the grief process.
Comprehension Level	
C2.1 Illustrates the stress-adaptation phenomenon.	Cite an example of a patient in stress and the adaptive response exhibited.
C2.2 Distinguishes between the behavior of integrity and that of despair in the elderly person.	Describe the behavior of the elderly person with a sense of integrity as it contrasts with that of the elderly person with a sense of despair.
C2.3 Makes inferences about the effect of air pollution on individuals with limited pulmonary function.	Predict the effects of smog on health of a person with emphysema.

BEHAVIORAL OBJECTIVES	TEST ITEM

Application Level

C3.0   Applies Erikson's crisis theory to the selection of appropriate nursing intervention.

Relate Erikson's crisis theory to the determination of the type of nursing intervention you would use in meeting the needs of parents with an acutely ill child.

Analysis Level

C4.1   Identifies assumptions underlying proposals for national health insurance.

Analyze one of the proposals for national health insurance and identify the assumptions underlying the major points in the plan.

C.4.2   Analyzes the relationship between the adolescent developmental level and societal pressures.

One county health department reported a marked increase in sexually transmitted disease among adolescents. How would you explain this phenomenon from the perspective of the relationship between the adolescent's developmental level and the pressures of society?

C4.3   Analyzes the form and pattern of a literary piece of work relevant to nursing.

Deduce the purpose, perspective, and feelings of the author in the book, *I Never Promised You a Rose Garden.*

Synthesis Level

C5.1   Writes an essay presenting a position on a health care issue.

Write an essay in which you present your reaction to the statement: Health is a human right.

C5.2   Proposes a plan of action for solving a problem within a health agency.

Write up a plan for combating institutional racism within a health agency.

C5.3   Formulates a conceptual scheme for categorizing nurse-patient interactions.

Devise a conceptual scheme for categorizing nurse-patient interactions in a family practice outpatient setting.

BEHAVIORAL OBJECTIVES	TEST ITEM
Evaluation Level C6.1 Makes judgments of a report of a nursing research project in terms of internal criteria.	Select a clinical nursing research report in *Nursing Research*. Evaluate the work in terms of internal criteria: logical accuracy, validity, reliability, precision of statements, logic of conclusions from data, and appropriate documentation.
C6.2 Evaluates a nursing research report in terms of external criteria.	Select a nursing research report from *Nursing Research*. Compare this report with another comparable report in the same area that is recognized as a valid and reliable study.

The following two examples suggest ways in which the essay form of question might be used to test in the affective domain:

A3.2 Examines various points of view on a controversial issue with the intent of declaring a position on it.	"Welfare patients admitted to a medical center hospital should expect to be used for medical research." 1. Identify two possible positions in regard to this statement. 2. Provide a rationale for each position. 3. Specify your stand on the issue inherent in this statement and support your choice.
A4.1 Forms judgments as to the constitutional rights of individuals admitted to a mental health care facility.	Using the Bill of Rights as a framework for your thinking, describe the constitutional rights of a person admitted to a mental health care facility.

One of the major limitations in the use of essay questions is that the sampling of content in a course is restricted. However, especially at the upper levels of the taxonomies, essay questions are particularly useful as out-of-class examinations. The questions used for testing at the synthesis and evaluation cognitive levels, presented as illustrations, are more suitable to out-of-class examinations because of their nature and scope. The questions illustrating evaluation in the affective domain may be used in either out-of-class or in-class situations.

PROBLEM-SOLVING EVALUATION

Problem-solving evaluation may be used as part of a pencil and paper test or given through computer-assisted instruction (CAI). It may be used for individual students or as an evaluation project for a group of students. In the latter instance, group members discuss the questions and present results of their deliberations in writing or orally to the rest of the class.

The use of problem-solving situations is designed to assess the student's ability for critical thinking. When this form of evaluation is used for clinical practice problem solving, students are presented with a clinical situation to be analyzed with the intent of identifying problems to be solved, deciding on actions to be taken, applying knowledge to a clinical problem, and clarifying own beliefs and values. When sufficient assessment data are presented in the case situation, questions can be asked to lead the student through the diagnostic reasoning process. Students also can be asked to identify and cluster cues from the assessment data; generate tentative hypotheses as to the nursing diagnoses, with supporting data; and decide upon the nursing diagnoses considering the alternatives proposed. Such an evaluation strategy provides information for both teacher and student as to ability to identify cues and generate hypotheses, both important components of the diagnostic reasoning process.

In problem-solving evaluation, the student may be presented with a written description of the problem situation and asked to respond to questions relative to it. The format of questions used in the situation may vary. One format, such as multiple recognition, may be used for all questions, or a variety of test items, such as multiple choice, essay, and alternate response, may be used.

Three types of test exercises are usually associated with this classification of evaluation: situation, critical incident, and decision-making. Problem situations expressed in any of these three types often test more than one behavioral objective per situation and may be used with any level of the cognitive and affective domains.

GENERAL PRINCIPLES OF CONSTRUCTION

1. The problem-solving situation should be geared to the learner's knowledge and experience.
2. Information about the incident or situation should be sufficient to assure clarity in the presentation.

3. The situation must be reasonable in length so that the learner is not required to devote a long period of time reading and rereading the description.

4. In a critical incident, the information should be described briefly with no extraneous material included.

5. Questions posed must be related directly to the data incorporated in the description.

Situation

The situation test, based on the cognitive-field theory of learning and theories of problem solving, describes a situation pertinent to nursing which incorporates all of the data significant to understanding the nature of the problem. Questions relate typically to the problem-solving process, components of the diagnostic reasoning process, nursing actions and related theory, or the theoretical basis for nursing practice, as indicated in the situation.

ILLUSTRATIONS

ILLUSTRATION 1

BEHAVIORAL OBJECTIVE

A3.1   Expresses own feelings about ways individuals respond to stress.

C4.1   Deduces stress factors in a patient-family situation.

C3.0   Applies theories of stress and coping to a clinical situation.

INSTRUCTIONS

Read the following situation and then answer the questions.

SITUATION

Ms. J, a 20-year old mother of three children, ranging in age from six months to three years, lives with her mother and younger brother in a three-room apartment in the city. Never married, Ms. J has been receiving assistance from Aid to Dependent Children since the birth of her first child.

During last evening, Ms. J was brought to the emergency unit of the hospital in acute distress from heroin overdose. She is now a patient on your unit, and you have been assigned to care for her.

QUESTIONS

1. What are your feelings about Ms. J as you prepare to plan her care?
2. What stressors do you identify in her life situation as described here?
3. Explain the dynamics of this patient-family situation on the basis of the Lazarus's stress and coping theory.
4. What is your opinion about the way Ms. J is handling her stressors?

ILLUSTRATION II

BEHAVIORAL OBJECTIVES

C4.2   Relates patient's reaction to impending death to the stage in the grief process being experienced.

C4.2   Responds to patient's concerns consistent with his reaction to impending death.

A4.1   Explores own values about death as they relate to the variables of age and cause of death.

INSTRUCTIONS

Read the following situation and then answer the questions according to the stated directions.

SITUATION

John, a 16-year-old, has leukemia and knows it. Readmitted to the hospital for the third time, now in critical condition, he says to the nurse, "It is good I had to come this time during summer vacation, so I am not going to waste any more time from school. You know, I'll graduate from high school in one year and I want to keep my A average to go straight to college. In this way it will not take me more than four years to become a lawyer since the doctors told me it doesn't look too good for me."

QUESTIONS

1. John's comments suggest that he is in the _____ stage of the grief process.
2. The mechanism by which John is handling the stress of dying is called _____.

Circle the letter that appears in front of the *one* statement that completes correctly the statement in questions 3 and 4.

3. If you were the nurse, your interpretation of John's statement would be:

   a. John has not understood the doctor's explanation about the fatal prognosis of his disease.

   b. John acts as a typical adolescent who is trying to impress you with his scholastic performance.

   c. John knows about his prognosis, but denies it.

   d. John knows about his prognosis, but bargains for the time left.

4. To help John progress through the grief process, the best response you could make to his comment would be:

   a. "Congratulations, John, I am glad to know that you are a good student."

   b. "Does it bother you that this disease might interfere with your studies, John?"

   c. "You are right, John, so you will be in good shape when school starts in September."

   d. "Don't worry about school now, John. The important thing is that you will be feeling better."

Circle the "A" before the following statements with which you agree; circle the "D" before the following statements with which you disagree; and circle the "U" before the following statements about which you are uncertain. Support your choice in the space provided.

5. A. U. D.   John's death from leukemia is more tragic than it would have been if his death occurred with a drug overdose.

6. A. U. D.   It is more tragic for John to die of leukemia than for a man of 60 to die from the same disease.

7. A. U. D.   John's comments suggest he is making an appropriate adaptation to the stress caused by his impending death.

ILLUSTRATION III

BEHAVIORAL OBJECTIVE

C4.2   Identifies possible diagnostic hypotheses based on data presented.

INSTRUCTIONS

Read the following situation and then answer the questions.

SITUATION

Mr. A is a 60 year-old patient who recently had a laryngectomy. His incision is healing and requires a dressing change once daily. He has been unable to sleep though for the past two nights because of pain in his neck radiating to his shoulder. Mr. A admits to having a "drinking problem" and long history of smoking. Over the past three years, he has lost significant amount of weight. Mr. A lives alone; he has been unemployed for the last three years. As you enter the room, Mr. A writes on his memo pad, "Please help me. I can't stand the pain anymore."

QUESTIONS

1. List possible hypotheses as to nursing diagnoses. Include all of the hypotheses to be considered.

2. For each hypothesis, describe supporting assessment data.

3. What additional data are needed, if any, to support or reject each hypothesis?

Critical Incident

Critical incident is the second form of evaluation suggested under the rubric of problem solving. It is a description of an event in which data are limited to factors that have a direct bearing on the event itself. Questions in this area generally relate to a nursing judgment and/or actions such as: assessment, interpretation of data, prediction of consequences, formulation of hypotheses, suggestions for intervention, or determination of criteria for evaluation.

ILLUSTRATIONS

ILLUSTRATION I

BEHAVIORAL OBJECTIVE

C2.2   Determines types of data appropriate for a nursing decision.

INSTRUCTIONS

Read the incident below and respond to the question.

CRITICAL INCIDENT

A nurse enters the room of a 45-year-old male to take his blood pressure as ordered. The nurse finds that the reading is 80/50, a drop from 100/80 at the reading four hours ago.

QUESTION

What questions should the nurse raise to focus the data collection necessary for determining the decision for action?

ILLUSTRATION II

BEHAVIORAL OBJECTIVES

A3.1 Examines own feelings about the elderly person's need to live a meaningful life.

C3.0 Uses relevant theories in interpreting the dynamics in a critical incident.

INSTRUCTIONS

Read the incident below and respond to the questions.

CRITICAL INCIDENT

Three months after the death of his wife of 52 years, you see Mr. A, an 81-year-old man, walking down the street holding hands with a female contemporary. They are laughing and appear happy.

QUESTIONS

1. What would be your initial reaction upon seeing Mr. A and his friend? Why do you react in this manner?

2. How does Mr. A's behavior relate to the Erikson concept of the age of integrity?

3. How do you really feel about Mr. A's behavior?

Decision Making

This form of question provides a description of a nursing action that involves a nursing decision. Three approaches to decision-making exercises may be used:

1. Describe a situation up to a point of decision. Ask the student to make the decision indicated and provide a rationale for the choice.

2. Describe a situation, including the decision. Ask the student to state agreement or disagreement with the decision and support the response.

3. Describe the situation, including the decision. Ask the student if the information provided is sufficient for a decision. If the response is in the negative, ask the student to indicate what other information is indicated.

In some instances 2 and 3 are combined.

The decision-making process involves identifying clues indicating that a decision is necessary, assessing the situation, selecting alternatives for action considering consequences of each action, establishing priority of choices, and evaluating the outcomes. This type of evaluation is especially important in helping the student develop divergent thinking ability, the process by which the student arrives at several alternative solutions. It is the requirement of the student's recognition of alternatives and the selection of the best of the alternatives that makes this type of test situation a particularly valuable evaluation strategy for determining the student's critical thinking competency.

ILLUSTRATIONS

ILLUSTRATION I

BEHAVIORAL OBJECTIVE

C3.0   Uses decision-making process in meeting the expressed needs of an individual.

INSTRUCTIONS

Read the situation below and respond to the questions.

DECISION-MAKING INCIDENT

Mr. P, a 48-year-old college professor, has inoperable cancer. No one has informed him of his diagnosis. One morning while you are providing care to him he states, "I wish someone would tell me what is wrong with me." You feel that his statement calls for a decision for action.

QUESTIONS

1. What clue(s) in the situation have convinced you that a decision is indicated?
2. What is your assessment of Mr. P's situation?
3. Identify three alternative courses of action that could be taken.
4. Describe the possible consequences of each course of action.
5. What decision would you select? Support your choice of decision.

ILLUSTRATION II

BEHAVIORAL OBJECTIVE

C4.2 Analyzes a decision for a nursing action from the perspective of the decision-making process.

INSTRUCTIONS

Read the situation below and respond to the questions accordingly.

DECISION-MAKING INCIDENT

A senior nursing student in a community health experience made a visit with the instructor. The purpose of the visit was the health supervision of a premature male infant now nine months old. It is the practice of the health department to follow premature infants for one year.

Mrs. Brown greeted the student warmly, stating that she was glad for the visit because her son, John, seemed to be ill. She stated, "He must have broken out during the night. He wasn't sick yesterday, why we even visited by next door neighbor. She's pretty excited because she thinks she's pregnant. She missed two periods."

The student examined the baby and noted a generalized rash and enlarged cervical nodes. Suspecting rubella, the student shared her findings with Mrs. Brown. She urged Mrs. Brown to take John to the physician for diagnosis and any necessary treatment.

QUESTIONS

1. What is the decision for action the nursing student made? Do you agree with it?

   Yes ⎯⎯⎯⎯⎯⎯ No ⎯⎯⎯⎯⎯⎯

2. Are the data sufficient for you as the nurse in this situation to make a decision?

   Yes ⎯⎯⎯⎯⎯⎯ No ⎯⎯⎯⎯⎯⎯

   If no, what other data would you need?

3. Analyze this situation in terms of each step of the decision-making process.

4. What decision would you make if you were the nursing student in this situation? Support your choice.

Problem-solving situations are designed to test levels of cognitive ability beyond the skill of recall. Nursing, as a practice discipline, *uses* knowledge. Therefore, evaluation procedures that call upon students to demonstrate competency in using knowledge are of particular significance. Problem-solving test strategies provide data that help to identify the theoretical base of the learner's actions, as distinct from intuitions or imitation. These test situations also help both the learner and teacher to be aware of values the learner holds and to assess these values as to their appropriateness to a practitioner in a helping profession.

MULTIMEDIA

The use of multimedia in educational programs has increased markedly during the past decade, but its use in evaluation has been limited. Multimedia increase the variety of senses, such as hearing, touching, and seeing images, used by the student during an evaluation experience. The increased sensory stimulation adds more depth in a test situation and increases the scope of evaluation. Multimedia are especially amenable to simulation testing.

In previous illustrations of problem-solving situations, there was sole reliance on the written word. If visual imagery and tonal qualities were added to the situations so that the learner could see the participants engaged in action and hear their conversations, then the whole evaluation experience would take on more dynamic dimensions and the student could become more involved in the process. If the student had been able to see Mr. A and his female companion, this direct contact may have elicited a more perceptive response than would be possible simply as a result of reading about the incident.

Multimedia may be used with other forms of evaluation. Questions may be posed in any of the formats previously discussed in this chapter. They may be used in in-class situations, although they are particularly effective for out-of-class exercises, especially where students have access to a learning laboratory. Many types of media may be used for projecting the test situations. The following suggestions are made for consideration in the use of films, videotapes, computers, audio tapes, slides, and pictures.

Films provide for visual and, in most cases, auditory stimulation. Added stimuli facilitate testing of students' problem-solving abilities and help in determining the values and beliefs upon which students base their actions. A film situation may depict events such as nursing action; patient behavior; individual, family, or group responses to phenomena in a setting; or action within an environment. They are particularly useful in critical-incident testing and decision-making testing.

Videotapes provide for visual and auditory stimulation and have a start-stop capability. Their use is similar to the use of films, except in instances where videotapes are made of the learner in a practice situation. In this instance, videotapes are an effective means of formative evaluation, for the learner and the teacher (and in some instances other learners) have the opportunity to appraise the learner's practice and analyze it critically.

Videotapes are particularly effective for simulation testing. A simulation creates an experience that represents a real-life situation. In a simulation, information relative to a nursing situation is presented to the learner who then makes decisions about some aspect of it. The simulation may be depicted in a videotape or presented by computer. In assisting students in the development of skill in diagnostic reasoning, a videotape may be used to present assessment data from which students then generate possible diagnostic hypotheses with supporting data. Such a strategy also may be used for evaluation of the student's ability in this area. Plunkett and Olivieri (1989) describe use of a videotape as part of a simulation teaching method designed to assist students in developing skill in the diagnostic reasoning process. They emphasize that the focus of the simulation is on generating hypotheses from the data and exploring each one instead of arriving at one correct hypothesis or stating a specific nursing diagnosis. Feedback from the teacher throughout the simulation and in the debriefing period makes this type of strategy appropriate particularly for formative evaluation.

In a computer simulation of a clinical problem or situation, the student responds to data presented by the computer, make a decision, and receives feedback on the consequences of that decision (Reilly & Oermann, 1985). Some computer programs are so designed that the client's status is altered by the decisions made which communicates vividly to students the outcomes of their decisions. This type of computer program is useful for formative evaluation since immediate feedback is given to the learner. In interactive video, the computer simulation is combined with a videotape, thus allowing the student to view the simulated situation in the videotape and respond to questions presented by the computer. Interactive video is also useful for formative evaluation since immediate feedback is provided based on the student's response. In addition, the learner has an opportunity to access video segments to clarify own answers (Battista-Calderone, 1989).

Audiotapes add an auditory dimension to the evaluation strategy. They can be used with illustrations of music, reading of literature, verbal interactions among or between individuals in group work, and various sounds, such as heart and lung. The tape recording approach may be used to assess a student's competency in interpreting or analyzing interviews, the client–nurse teaching situations, the group process, or an individual's expression of ideas, beliefs, or values. In the teaching of physical assessment skills, evaluation of the learner's ability to discriminate body sounds may be assisted by the tape recording strategy. When tapes are used in conjunction with slides or film-strips, visual stimulation is added, and topics used for evaluation can be extended to problem-solving situations, as described for films.

Slides and pictures provide for visual imagery. They may be used in atti-tude testing, for example, when a student is requested to interpret the mean-ing of the scene depicted. They may also serve as an important means of assessing the student's ability to make critical judgments relative to the "rightness" or "wrongness" of some aspect portrayed. This type of judgment may relate to such images as the method of holding an infant, methods for positioning patients, the positioning of a nurse while carrying out a specific action, or the characteristics of an environment. A series of slides may repre-sent steps in a process that may be interpreted or critically analyzed by the learner.

GENERAL PRINCIPLES OF CONSTRUCTION

1. Selection of the appropriate multimedia device must be determined by the behavioral objective.

2. Unless the learner has access to the equipment used for the test situation for repeated viewing or listening, the situation for the test should be short enough (about 1–3 minutes) for the student to remember.

3. Behaviors to be evaluated as well as the test question should be presented to the student before the testing begins so that the stu-dent is able to focus attention on significant aspects.

4. Questions can relate only to the events depicted in the situation.

5. When visual imagery is used in class situations, all students must have a clear and unobstructed view.

ILLUSTRATIONS

ILLUSTRATION OF TAPE RECORDING

BEHAVIORAL OBJECTIVE

C4.1   Differentiates the sounds elicited when percussion technique is used.

INSTRUCTIONS

Listen to the tape recording, "Sounds in Percussion," and answer the following questions.

QUESTIONS

1. Identify the different percussion sounds recorded on the tape.
2. Describe the differentiating characteristics of each sound.
3. Identify a location in the body where each type of sound may be heard.

ILLUSTRATION OF SLIDES AND TAPE RECORDING

BEHAVIORAL OBJECTIVES

C2.2 Distinguishes the stereotyped comments made by the nurse.

C3.0 Chooses two alternative approaches the nurse could have used in greeting the client.

C2.1 Cites examples of own stereotyped responses in handling anxiety.

INSTRUCTIONS

View the single-concept slide series and listen to the accompanying tape for "Interactions for Study." Respond to the questions accordingly.

(This vignette depicts a nurse conversing with a patient who has had a C.V.A. While exercising the patient's affected arm, the nurse responds to the patient's expressed concerns in a trite and nonlistening manner.)

QUESTIONS

1. Identify at least two stereotypic comments made by the nurse during this interaction.
2. Write two alternate approaches the nurse could use to convey her interest and concern for how Mrs. Bolin is feeling. Explain how the approaches you suggest differ from those in the slide/tape recording.
3. Describe an incident in which you have felt anxious while interacting with a client. What stereotypic responses did you give in that situation?

ILLUSTRATION OF THE USE OF A FILM

BEHAVIORAL OBJECTIVE

C4.1 Identifies the nursing functions of the clinic nurse in meeting the needs of the pregnant woman.

INSTRUCTIONS

View the section of the film, *A World of Contrasts: A Time of Hope*, which portrays the visit of a pregnant woman to the clinic, and then respond to the questions.

(This film has six separate episodes, each portraying a concept of community health nursing. The episode used for this testing shows primarily a young pregnant woman and a clinic nurse in interaction, although there are a few views of a parent-teaching class.)

QUESTIONS

In the film, a pregnant woman comes to the clinic for prenatal care.

1. What nursing functions are identified as the responsibility of the nurse in this situation?

2. Are you satisfied that the functions identified are compatible with the concept of primary care nursing?

   Yes _____ No _____

   If not, what changes or additions would you suggest based on the concept of primary care nursing in this type of health care setting?

Multimedia add sensory dimensions to the evaluation process and have the potential for involving the learner who is called upon more and more to respond to a greater variety of sensory stimuli.

PAPERS AND OTHER WRITTEN ASSIGNMENTS

Written work provides teachers with an excellent opportunity to assess the student's ability relative to the thinking process, the communication of ideas, and the values and beliefs operant. (Some of the written work is more relevant to clinical practice and will be discussed in a later chapter.) Critical analysis of readings, phenomena or situations, essays, defense of positions on issues, and reports of studies can follow the patterns previously illstrated. Many of the suggestions for questions stated in the essay section are particularly pertinent. Further illustrative examples will not be given, but some general principles are offered.

GENERAL PRINCIPLES

1. The behavioral objective(s) for the assignment must be stated clearly.
2. Instructions must be stated clearly and understood by the learner.

3. Provision should be made for individual guidance as the need is indicated, so that the student can aspire to mastery.

4. Learners should be notified of standards for evaluation and the basis for grading.

5. Faculty should support creative approaches to meeting objectives.

6. Written work deviating from the prescribed format should be assessed in terms of its response to the objectives, not its adherence to an expected form.

GROUP PROJECTS

Evaluation of individual performance causes less concern for teachers than evaluation of an individual in a group activity. The question arises as to whether or not all individuals in a group should receive the same evaluation and perhaps the same grade. Questions relate to equity in the quality of each member's participation. If there is no equity, the teacher must decide what measures are just and fair for discriminating differences. Evaluation of a group project should provide opportunity for assessing the group as a whole as well as individual performance within the group.

GENERAL PRINCIPLES

1. As with any evaluation procedure, group activities are directed toward achieving behavioral objectives on which the group will be evaluated.

2. Faculty and students participate in determining behaviors that will be used to evaluate the group.

3. Behaviors include those appropriate to the substance of the report as well as to standards of communication.

4. The evaluation also provides for comments that evidence discrimination among the participants' attainment of the behaviors.

5. There must be provision for process as well as outcome evaluation.

6. Group members evaluate each other's participation in the group.

7. When group presentation is given before a class or a similar group, all viewers of the presentation participate in the evaluation.

8. When group presentation is given before a class or a similar group, the evaluation form is completed immediately after the presentation while the perception of the process is clear in the minds of the evaluators.

ILLUSTRATION—GROUP
PRESENTATION BEFORE A CLASS

Figure 8-1 illustrates a form that was used to evaluate the performance of a group of students who presented a project for the course *Perspectives in Nursing*. The content behaviors are those designed for the project. This form, developed by students and faculty, was completed by participants in the group as well as by members of the class, and was submitted at the conclusion of each group's presentation. Data were analyzed and a profile for each group was determined as well as a content analysis on items III and IV.

Figure 8-2 shows the second evaluation form used in the project. As with the previous form, this was developed jointly by faculty and students, and each participant in the presenting group completed a self-evaluation and also evaluated colleagues in the group. The focus was to assist the assessment of each member as to performance during the developmental process of the project. Data were analyzed and a profile made for each of the participants.

These examples illustrate forms which may be developed for evaluating the total group presentation as well as the participation of each member in the group.

ILLUSTRATION—SEMINAR

In a seminar, another group activity, the issues of evaluation are different from the group project described above. The student participates as a leader and as a contributing member at various times throughout the seminar.

Figure 8-3 is an illustration of the behaviors identified by a group of graduate students in a seminar course. Each member evaluated every other member of the group. The procedure identifies four major variables— leadership role in the seminar, quality of the content of the presentation, quality of the presentation, and the participant role. Students identified behaviors expected under each heading and used them to write a descriptive evaluation of each other at the end of the course. It might be noted that the

EVALUATION OF GROUP PROJECT

Topic:
Date:
Participants:

Behavioral objectives relative to the presentation of reports are listed below. Opposite each behavioral objective is a scale representing the degree of attainment. *Circle the number* on the scale which you feel best represents the group's attainment of the objective.

I. *Content*

1. Defines the issue.   (not attained) 1 2 3 4 5 6 (attained)

2. Describes the present state of the issue including supportive and constraining factors.   (not attained) 1 2 3 4 5 6 (attained)

3. Discriminates elements which make it an issue.   (not attained) 1 2 3 4 5 6 (attained)

4. Describes the meaning of the issue to nursing and to society.   (not attained) 1 2 3 4 5 6 (attained)

5. Deduces the origin of the issue.   (not attained) 1 2 3 4 5 6 (attained)

6. Describes the status of the issue within the context of society at particular periods of time.   (not attained) 1 2 3 4 5 6 (attained)

7. Identifies role of particular individuals who had a significant impact on the issue throughout its course.   (not attained) 1 2 3 4 5 6 (attained)

8. Predicts the state of the issue in the future.   (not attained) 1 2 3 4 5 6 (attained)

9. Presents a hypothesis for the future.   (not attained) 1 2 3 4 5 6 (attained)

10. Provides rationale for hypothesis.   (not attained) 1 2 3 4 5 6 (attained)

11. Identifies changes necessary for the future prediction.   (not attained) 1 2 3 4 5 6 (attained)

II. *Method of Presentation*

1. Organizes presentation in a clear, logical manner.   (not attained) 1 2 3 4 5 6 (attained)

2. Communicates ideas clearly.   (not attained) 1 2 3 4 5 6 (attained)

3. Evidences continuity among presenters.   (not attained) 1 2 3 4 5 6 (attained)

4. Makes provisions for discussion by class members.   (not attained) 1 2 3 4 5 6 (attained)

5. Responds to questions in a knowledgeable manner.   (not attained) 1 2 3 4 5 6 (attained)

6. Shows originality in the presentation.   (not attained) 1 2 3 4 5 6 (attained)

III. *General Comments*

IV. *Comments Regarding Specific Participants*

Figure 8–1
Sample Form for Evaluation of Group Project

EVALUATION OF INDIVIDUAL PARTICIPATION

Name of Participant:
Topic of Group:

Rate each of the five behaviors listed below, circle the appropriate numbers, and support your position in the space provided.

1. Assumes responsibility for own share of the work.   (Little) 1 2 3 4 5 6 7 (Much)
   COMMENT:

2. Helps rest of the group in getting resources.   (Little) 1 2 3 4 5 6 7 (Much)
   COMMENT:

3. Willingly shares ideas with colleagues.   (Little) 1 2 3 4 5 6 7 (Much)
   COMMENT:

4. Brings new ideas to the group.   (Little) 1 2 3 4 5 6 7 (Much)
   COMMENT:

5. Shares leadership, responsibility.   (Little) 1 2 3 4 5 6 7 (Much)
   COMMENT:

6. Other comments.

Figure 8–2
Sample Form for Evaluation of Individual Participation

same form was used to evaluate the faculty member, who was considered a seminar member and responsible for presenting one of the seminars. The evaluations were summarized for each student.

Evaluation of group projects must provide opportunity to gather data on individual as well as on group performance. This involves student-teacher participation in determining behaviors as well as in the process itself. In addition to obtaining a data base for evaluative judgment, this approach also enables the student to gain experience in self-evaluation and in the evaluation of others.

Seminar in Nursing Education
EVALUATION

Name: SEMINAR Member:

1. Leadership Role in Seminar
    Shares leadership responsibility with colleagues.
    Modifies plan when indicated on the basis of analysis of group dynamics.
    Supports participants in their efforts to be active in the group process.
    Provides for freedom of thought and expression of all participants.
    Helps the group synthesize ideas presented.

2. Quality of Content of Presentation
    Prepares objectives which encourage an analytic approach.
    Proposes readings which are relevant to the objectives.
    Develops content on an appropriate theoretical basis.
    Relates content to stated objectives.
    Analyzes issues in terms of their relationship to society, the profession, and self.
    Analyzes issues in terms of past, present, and future dimensions.

3. Quality of Presentation
    Organizes material in a clear manner.
    Explains material in a clear, comprehensive manner.
    Utilizes methods appropriate to presentation.
    Plans presentation so as to allow for group participation.
    Clarifies points when indicated.

4. Participant Role in Seminar
    Supports viewpoints with rationale.
    Contributes to the discussion in a scholarly fashion.
    Willingly shares ideas and feelings with colleagues.
    Respects right of all individuals to agree/disagree with one's opinion.
    Is able to agree/disagree with idea without attacking individual.
    Uses intellectual discipline in handling disagreement.
    Analyzes effect of self on group process.

Figure 8–3
Sample Form for Seminar Evaluation

SUMMARY

There is a direct relationship between the *what* and the *how* of evaluation. Evaluation strategies must be appropriate to specified behavior.

In any educational endeavor, it is important that a variety of strategies be prepared to meet the individual needs of leaners and the particular nature of the situation. Efforts must be made to direct evaluation at the cognitive level beyond that of recall, for nurses must be able to demonstrate competency in their use of knowledge in a variety of circumstances. Evaluation must also include strategies for determining the affective as well as the cognitive level of development, for values are determinants of behavior.

Use of the taxonomies in defining expected behavior is helpful in stating the level desired. It is essential, however, that the evaluation procedure be designed in such a way as to be compatible with the specified behavior. Various strategies include: paper and pencil tests (alternate response, multiple recognition, completion, matching, and essay); problem solving (situation, critical incident, and decision making); multimedia; papers and other written work; and group projects.

REFERENCES

Battista-Calderone, A. (1989). Designing interactive video instruction. *Nursing & Health Care, 10*(9), 505–510.

Plunkett, E. J., & Olivieri, R. J. (1989). A strategy for introducing diagnostic reasoning: Hypothesis testing using a simulation approach. *Nurse Educator, 14*(16), 27–31.

Reilly, D. E., & Oermann, M. H. (1985) *The clinical field: Its use in nursing education.* Norwalk, CT: Appleton-Century-Crofts.

RECOMMENDED READINGS

Belfry, M. J., & Winne, P. H. (1988). A review of the effectiveness of computer assisted instruction in nursing education. *Computers in Nursing, 6*(2), 77–85.

Brundenell, I., & Carpenter, C. S. (1990). Adult learning styles and attitudes toward computer assisted instruction. *Journal of Nursing Education, 29*(2), 79–83.

Burns, K. A. (1984). Experience in the use of gaming and simulation as an evaluation tool for nurses. *Journal of Continuing Education in Nursing, 15*(5), 213–217.

Cassidy, V. R. (1987). Response changing and student achievement on objective tests. *Journal of Nursing Education, 26*(2), 60–62.

Cassidy, V. R. (1987). Test construction techniques. *Journal of Nursing Staff Development, 3*(4), 154–158.

Chang, B. L. (1986). Computer-aided instruction in nursing education. In H.H. Werley, J.J. Firzpatrick, & R.L. Taunton (Eds.), *Annual review of nursing research* (pp. 217–233). New York: Springer.

Chenevey, B. (1988). Constructing multiple-choice examinations: Item writing. *Journal of Continuing Education in Nursing, 19*(5), 201–204.

Clayton, G. M., & Broome, M. (1989). *Instruments for use in nursing education research.* New York: National League for Nursing.

Ebel, R. L., & Frisbie, D. A. (1986). *Essentials of educational measurement* (4th ed.). Englewood Cliffs, NJ: Prentice-Hall.

Gronlund, N. E., & Linn, R. L. (1990). *Measurement and evaluation in teaching* (6th ed.). New York: Macmillan.

Hopkins, C. D., & Antes, R. L. (1985). *Classroom measurement and evaluation* (2nd ed.). Itasca, IL: F.E. Peacock.

Hopkins, K. D., Stanley, J. C., & Hopkins, B. R. (1990). *Educational and psychological measurement and evaluation* (7th ed.). Englewood Cliffs, NJ: Prentice-Hall.

Litwack, L., Linc, L., & Bower, D. (1985). *Evaluation in nursing: Principles and practice.* New York: National League for Nursing.

Nichols, E. G., & Miller, G. K. (1984). Interreader agreement on comprehensive essay examinations. *Journal of Nursing Education, 23*(2), 64–69.

Oermann, M. H. (1984). An instrument for analyzing curriculum materials in nursing. *Journal of Nursing Education, 23,* 404–406.

Oermann, M. H. (1984). Analyzing and selecting audio-visual materials. *Nurse Educator, 9*(4), 24–27.

Oermann, M. H. (1990). Research on teaching methods. In G.M. Clayton & P.A. Baj (EDS.), *Review of research in nursing education* (pp. 1–31). New York: National League for Nursing.

Rickelman, B., Taylor-Fox, J., Reisch, J., Payne, P., & Jelemensky, L. (1988). Effect of a CVIS instructional program regarding therapeutic communication on student learning and anxiety. *Journal of Nursing Education, 27*(7), 312–320.

Schleutermann, J. A., Holzemer, W. L., & Farrand, L. L. (1983). An evaluation of paper-and-pencil and computer-assisted simulations. *Journal of Nursing Education, 22*(8), 315–323.

Schneider, H. (1984). *Effective test construction in the health professions.* Jackson, MS: H. and B. Hess Co.

Stedman, C. H. (1985). Testing for competence: Lessons from health professions. *The Educational Forum, 49*(2), 199–210.

Summers, S., Hoffman, J., Neff, E. J., Hanson, S., & Pierce, K. (1990). The effects of 60 beats per minute music on test taking anxiety among nursing students. *Journal of Nursing Education, 29*(2), 66–70.

Tripp, A., & Tollefson, N. (1985). Are complex multiple-choice options more difficult and discriminating than conventional multiple-choice options? *Journal of Nursing Education, 24*(3), 92–98.

Vallerand, A. H. (1988). Differences in test performance and learner satisfaction among nurses with varying autonomy levels. *Journal of Continuing Education in Nursing, 19*(5), 216–222.

Van Ort, S. (1989). Evaluating audio-visual and computer programs for classroom use. *Nurse Educator, 14*(1), 16–18.

Van Ort, S., & Hazzard, M. E. (1985). A guide for evaluation of test items. *Nurse Educator, 10*(5), 13–15.

Waltz, C. F., & Miller, C. H. (Eds.). (1988). *Educational outcomes: Assessment of quality —A compendium of measurement tools for baccalaureate nursing programs.* New York: National League for Nursing.

9

Test Construction

What will be on the test? Will we be responsible for this on our final? What will the exam cover? Do these questions sound familiar? How often do faculty hear students raise these questions before examination time? Why are these questions being raised? What are students really saying?

The students' questions are really symptomatic of a serious malady of the testing process and its relationship to the total educational endeavor.

TESTING PROCESS

Eble (1976) suggests that there are three crucial questions faculty must ask relative to the testing of students: (1) Why am I testing? (2) How am I testing? (3) What results am I getting?

Why Am I Testing?

The system of testing that a teacher uses influences to a marked degree the quality of student learning that occurs, the substance of the learning, and the study habits of students. Bigge (1982), Lowman, (1984), Milton, Pollio, and Eison (1986). The student's perception of what is worth knowing as a result of the learning experiences is what is on the test.

Each teacher needs to ponder very carefully the response to the question, Why am I testing? Testing is often acclaimed as a valuable component of the learning process. Lowman (1984) affirms this position, "A thoughtfully constructed examination can actually teach by stimulating students to think about concepts in new ways, notice new relationships and come to different insights" (pp. 187–188).

The student questions referred to at the beginning of this chapter suggest, however, that often students have experiences in testing that have not been perceived as growth-directed, but rather a process of checking to see "if they have learned." Some faculty practices may have prompted this image such as unannounced quizzes, unexpected material being tested, and emphasis on testing trivia.

A further factor precipitating these questions from students is the general practice of awarding grades on tests. Grades do have a significant influence on the student's progression in the program and even have a societal value which may affect career options. Students vary in their response to grades as a motivating factor, however. Milton et al. (1986) found that students who are high-learning/low-grade oriented score high in facilitative anxiety which enables them to meet the challenge of learning via tests with anxious anticipation. High-grade/low-learning students have high debilitating anxiety in test situations usually accompanied by poor study skills and concrete thinking. These students have a survival orientation to testing and approach tests in terms of their perception of what the teacher wants.

The issue of test anxiety must be considered by the teacher. Most teachers recognize that testing for many individuals is an anxiety-producing experience, some facilitative and some debilitative. Research into the phenomenon of test anxiety continues. Symptoms of worry, emotionality, and physical disturbances are recognized. Anxious students often encounter cognitive interference during tests so that negative personal thoughts interfere with the encoding, organization, and retrievability of information. Barnes (1987) studied this problem with a group of graduate nursing students involved in comprehensive examinations. The findings indicated a significant correlation between general test anxiety, pretest anxiety (worry and emotionality), and cognitive interference. Phillips' (1988) study of baccalaureate nursing students' anxiety at testing time indicated that test anxiety is multidimensional with cognitive interference associated more closely with academic self-concept than with study habits or test-taking skills. Benjamin et al. (1981) pose the notion that the worry that many students evidence at test time is due to lack of knowledge of content rather than to any individual traits.

Testing practices can aggravate test anxiety and foster cynicism on the part of students. Do teachers see testing as a strategy for maintaining control of the learning situation? The warning to the student, "You had better know this material for it will be on the test," is not an infrequent occurrence, especially if a student elects to be absent from the classroom session. One cannot deny the power disparity between student and faculty. The way the teacher uses that power is a major factor in the student's perception of the testing process.

But need tests be so threatening and detrimental to the pursuit of learning? Is there not a human need "to know what I know?" How many individuals enjoy doing crossword puzzles, answering quizzes that appear in popular magazines, or vicariously responding to questions on television programs? It is this basic need "to know what I know" that is diminished by our present education practices. In the educational system, the need to know is often not for the pure joy and satisfaction of the pursuit of self-knowledge, but rather for survival.

Testing is important and has a significant role in the educational process. Its feedback provides much data which have the potential for contributing to student and teacher growth, as well as the development of the program. The diagnostic function of a test is most significant, yet this practice is not used to its potential. Indeed the diagnostic value is ignored in courses that primarily emphasize the final examination, for by the time the test is given, the student's opportunities to redress the difficulties have ceased.

Tests can be used for both formative and summative evaluation purposes. It is essential that the teacher clearly define which of these purposes is basic to the particular test. One must remember that summative evaluation is also diagnostic, but the diagnosis is concerned with future learning, not the current one in which the student has been participating.

Used within a systematic formative and summative evaluation protocol, testing is most important in helping the student know what knowledge has been acquired and where there has been failure in understanding or in achieving competency. The teacher in such a process is able to determine the degree to which the objectives are achieved. The effectiveness of the teaching is also revealed since students indicate what they have learned or what they have not learned or understood.

How Am I Testing?

The question, How am I testing?, addresses two factors: the substance of the test and the testing strategies employed.

The substance of tests is often a source of great irritation and mistrust for students. One hears many complaints about the testing of trivia. Bruner (1963) addresses the issue of trivia testing as he discusses the structure of a discipline.

His comment regarding material worth knowing is paraphrased for nursing education. "Whether when fully developed as practitioners the subject or material is worth a graduate nurse's knowing and whether having known it as a student makes a person a better graduate nurse" (p. 52). Bruner challenges the educator to sort out the essentials from the trivia in teaching. Testing should be directed toward the essentials.

How are these essentials identified for both the teacher and the learner? The statement of behavioral objectives clearly denotes the subject matter to be learned and the behavior the student is expected to achieve in relation to this subject matter. Course unit examinations and quizzes are based on predetermined objectives so that both teacher and learner know the focus of the evaluation. The student's need to outguess what the teacher wants is incompatible with sound testing principles. The process for selecting testable content from the objectives is described later in this chapter.

The search for objective examinations is in vain, although individuals do often refer to *objective examinations*. The latter suggests certain formats that are readily scored and limit the options the responder has in answering the questions.

The subjective element is inherent in their very choice and, except for those addressed to known facts, the items often reflect the bias or the cultural values of the designers. The existence of the culturally biased test items which limit the use of many tests with certain populations is an established fact. The criterion of *fairness* is perhaps more realistic than a criterion of *objective*.

Regardless of the test format, fair questions can be developed which enable the student to discover what has been learned. One aspect of fairness relates to the student's understanding of the behavior to be tested. An objective that charges the student to develop the ability to *analyze* a phenomenon and demonstrate that competency in an evaluation situation does not permit the teacher to evaluate the ability to *recall* five components of the phenomenon. In other words, the testing strategy used and the question asked must be compatible with the behavior stated in the objective. If the students know beforehand the nature of the subject matter and the behavior to be demonstrated, then the student can approach the testing situation with a considerable degree of confidence. The energy needed to psych out the teacher and to try to determine what the student is expected to know for the test is instead expended toward needs relative to achievement on the test.

The question, How am I testing?, suggests another area of concern to faculty. This concern relates to the format used by faculty. How much variety in test design appears in the tests offered? Evidence suggests that faculty tend to get into a rut with many of these testing practices. They use the same general format each time. The end result is a test situation that is boring;

teachers are bored and students are bored. There is no excitement, but only boredom resulting from predictability and redundancy.

Lowman (1984) is concerned about the tendency of some teachers to offer the same testing format throughout the school term. Here, there is no accommodation for differences in students' preference for type of test, or in the measuring of objectives for different levels of knowledges and skills: recall, explanatory, or reflective. Milton et al. (1986) report that studies in the literature document that the majority of test questions in undergraduate courses, especially those with fixed responses such as multiple choice and true-false, seek simple factual information. The authors conducted a study of college student preferences regarding types of test questions and found that 81 percent of students preferred multiple choice because they were perceived to be easier, students could do better, and they could get better grades. The 19 percent who chose essay, a free response form of questioning, perceived this format as a means for learning and retaining the information more easily. Those students preferring essay questions were primarily from the high-learning/low-grade orientation group. The small number choosing essay questions may also be a function of their limited use in college.

Meyers (1986) believes that writing is one of the best means of processing, consolidating, and internalizing new knowledge. It is an important testing method for critical thinking because the outcome is visible and the teacher can see the student's thought as it develops.

Because nursing practice entails use of knowledge, it is this dimension rather than recall that must be tested. Professional practice requires reflective level thinking. Bigge (1982) supports writing as the best way to test at this intellectual level and thus recommends essay as the appropriate format. He states, "When we are teaching at a reflective level, one should be trying in testing as well as in all other evaluation procedures to ascertain whether each student is able to apply adequate information to the solution of the problem so as to harmonize the problem, all available data or facts, and the answer" (p. 340). Other forms of free response questions could meet the same evaluation criteria.

What Results Am I Getting?

The third question, What results am I getting?, is closely allied to the two preceding questions. The expectation of results is determined by the reason for testing and the process of testing. Unfortunately, some faculty look at testing as a form of triage, with the results often confirming prejudgments. However, for most faculty, the results serve the function of diagnostic feedback mentioned earlier. The results not only provide data about the performance of individual students, but they provide the teacher with some awareness of a class norm. Plans for assessing the results need to be carefully designed prior to the examination following the practice done with all other aspects of the test development.

TEST DEVELOPMENT

Although it is acknowledged that in our present educational society testing is often perceived as a threat to the ego and a detriment to self-development, it is also acknowledged that testing has a significant role in our educational process. The deterrent is not from testing itself, but rather from the misuse of the process. As an analogy, automobiles are important in our life style. They are not a menace in themselves, but rather become a menace as they are misused. The goal is to develop and use tests to serve as a facilitating process in nursing education, not as a deterrent.

Purpose

Two major approaches to testing the achievement of the student are available, and it is essential that the teacher determine which approach will be used in the examination being prepared. The development of test items and the interpretation of results are dependent upon this choice.

A *norm-referenced test* is developed with the intent of comparing a student's achievement in relation to that of the student's classmates or peer group. A relative standard is used in interpreting the results—the standard being the average performance of a group. Test data are analyzed from the perspective of the normal curve. Standardized tests are the most common example of this approach to testing.

A *criterion-referenced test* is developed with the intent of comparing a student's achievement in relation to performance standards. An absolute standard is used in interpreting results—the standard being acceptably defined prior to the testing situation. This form of testing is compatible with the concept of mastery of learning and highlights the student's attainment of the objectives of a program in relation to specific criteria. It is the testing approach most applicable to most testing events within a nursing program, especially since competency is a critical outcome.

The planning for the testing program of each course should consider the purpose of the particular test. Is the test to provide data about the student's performance according to the absolute or the relative standard? Are the test results to be used primarily for formative or summative evaluation? Not all tests should be administered for the purpose of grading. Are the tests designed to determine student achievement in the cognitive and the affective domains, or is only one domain to be tested?

There are other reasons for testing than the primary one of determining competency. Some tests may be designed to discriminate types of competency among various classifications of learners. Sometimes a test will be administered to acquaint the student with a certain format of testing. There is in reality a state of being *test wise*, the situation where a test result may reflect more an individual's skill in test-taking than competency in the subject matter the test is designed to measure.

There are multiple purposes for testing. It is important that the test designer know the purpose(s) for the test being prepared and that the students are also clear as to the purpose. The purpose, however, must take into account the other types of evaluative data being collected on the student. Since all evaluation is designed to assess competency of the student, there must be a relationship among all data generated by the various strategies. A test by itself will not be sufficient as the only evaluative strategy.

Planning

The following scenario is seen all too frequently in schools of nursing as tests are prepared.

> *It is less than a week before the final examination is to be administered. In a small conference room in a school of nursing, four faculty can be observed around the table. On the table are some open textbooks, copies of previous examinations, and lecture notes. Conversation goes as follows: "Shall we ask them this in the exam?" "Was this covered in class?" "How about using this question again since everyone ought to know this?" "They were all supposed to read this chapter, let's ask a question from this chapter"—End of this scenario.*

The scene, faculty preparing a final examination, now needs some analysis. How many errors are identifiable in this scene? Errors:

1. Time for planning was too close to examination.
2. Focus of the examination had no direction. It reflected a concept of teaching as telling and suggested a recall testing process.
3. No objectives for the course were evident to guide the test makers in the selection of content and testing strategy.

4. There was a suggestion of using this examination as a means of checking to see if students did their assignment.
5. The conversation evidenced the "they and us" syndrome. Students were never referred to as students, but always in the form of third person plural.

Unfortunately, the process of test development first presented is all too common. Test preparation is generally an "add on" activity with little evidence of careful planning, yet its use for influencing the life and careers of students is awesome. Planning for testing is integrated into the total planning process of each course or unit. Not only the placement of the testing within the course framework should be identified, but also the development of each test should be as carefully processed as is the content and all learning activities. In reality, the testing should be prepared before the course is even taught. If testing is used to determine the achievement of the student relative to the objective, then the testing can be developed once the objectives have been stated. Testing is not dependent upon what is covered in class, for learning occurs through many types of experiences.

Once rationale for the various testing periods within a course has been determined, it is essential that the time frame allocated to each testing period be designated. The time frame will be determined by the purpose and will have some influence on the sampling of behaviors to be tested and the strategies to be used.

The planning for the testing and the identification of its purpose within the total educational endeavor makes it imperative that appropriate tests be devised. Lenberg (1979) suggests three concepts that are critical to the development of appropriate tests for performance evaluation. These three concepts—(1) content, (2) characteristics, and (3) structure and process—provide a framework for test construction as well.

Selection of Content

Content relates to the subject matter of the test and the desired behavior the student is to exhibit. In written tests, the behavior is primarily cognitive. Affective behaviors can be tested at a lower level by suggesting a value preference behavior in response to a situation and at a higher level by requiring the student to respond cognitively to the rationale behind the behavior. The patterning behavior essential for validating true value commitment would be evaluated by methods other than testing.

The specification of areas emanate from the objectives which are stated.

These objectives must be appropriate to the level of the student and representative of the total array of designated areas of knowledge which can be reasonably expected of the student within that course at the particular time designated for the tests. The process for identifying testable content in an objective is described below. The following is a course objective.

At the conclusion of the course, the student will relate psychosocial concepts to the assessment process of individuals with minimal adaptive needs.

1. AREA TO BE TESTED.

The area to be tested in this objective is:

The relationship between psychosocial concepts and the assessment process.

2. DEFINITION.

The area to be tested within the expected knowledge must be given precise meaning. The precision specifies the types of patient problems to be addressed and the critical elements or test units to be tested. This definition of the area clarifies the limits of inclusion or exclusion and demands that the definition be stated simply and clearly.

Definition of area: psychosocial concepts relevant to the assessment of patients with minimal adaptive needs.

3. CRITICAL ELEMENTS.

The writing of the critical elements or test units derived from the definition of the area calls for behaviors that must be judged in the test. The level of behaviors is specified as acceptable to students at that particular time in their education when the test is administered. These elements or units represent those areas required by all students and the range of acceptability needs to be stated. They must be meaningful, significant, learnable, and centers of concentration and mastery.

It is advisable that a few critical elements or test units for each area be identified so that the emphasis can be addressed to the essentials.

Critical Elements or Test Units

Behavioral: demonstrate relationship

Psychosocial concepts related to minimal adaptive needs:

antecedent psychological and sociological events

present psychological and sociological events

    interpersonal actions and meanings

    psychosocial stressors

    psychosocial adaptation

Content then is addressed to the essentials in nursing practice appropriate to the developmental stage of the student when the test is scheduled. It calls for careful delineation of the critical elements or test units in the area specified by the objectives with those elements expected in the practice of the nurse. The adherence to this last suggestion, behaviors expected by all nursing students, may not be a prerequisite in tests which are designed to discriminate among students in terms of cognitive skills and handling of subject matter. Discriminating tests are norm referenced.

Characteristics

Characteristic concepts of test preparation refer to matters such as sampling, objectivity, acceptability, and comparability. *Sampling* is concerned with the most frequently encountered areas of nursing care. Questions need to reflect the usual type of nursing action within the framework of the course, not the unusual or esoteric which is out of the province of most students' experience.

In place of *objectivity*, the term *fair* could be substituted. The careful delineation from the objectives of areas of knowledge and the selection of critical elements or test units should provide questions addressed to essentials that are inherent in the practice of nursing.

Acceptability relates to the expectation of passing if the level is achieved. The baseline is the identification of the critical element or test unit when specified as the basis of nursing practice. Acceptability is defined in terms of practice and theory.

Comparability relates to the nature of the test items on tests so that each one calls for the same degree of complexity and demand on the student. In tests where students are provided with choice of test items, this comparability criterion is most important.

Structure and Process

Structure and process relate to the characteristics of consistency, flexibility, and availability of feedback. The concern of *consistency* relates to consistency among evaluators as well as consistency in the administering of tests. Every effort must be made to assure that there is consistency in interpreting each test. The definition of critical elements or test units with the clearly delineated boundaries of acceptability should be helpful. When there are many evaluators of test items for free-response questions, it is advisable that the same person evaluate all student responses on a particular question.

Consistency in the administration of a test is also important, for students need to know the expectations of their behavior during the test situation. Confusion abounds when some faculty in a school proctor tests while other faculty provide no monitoring or supervision. The practice of making available a person to clarify questions during the examination also varies among teachers and creates unnecessary tension and stress for students.

Consistency also relates to the pattern of providing instructions to students relative to their responsibility in responding to questions and their approach to answering the questions. There need not be consistency in test format; as a matter of fact, such a practice would be most destructive to the educational endeavor. However, the student can expect that the instructions will be clearly stated, thereby eliminating the question of whether it is better to guess and answer all questions or to omit questions and answer only those that the student can answer comfortably. The methods of scoring needs to be conveyed to the student on a consistent basis, so that the student can determine the best use of time during the examination process.

Flexibility, the other characteristic of the process, relates to the structure of the test. In a test situation, one can often feel a sense of being confined, with no perceived option to express self or "show what I know." Examinations that provide for choice often give the student some sense of control over the test situation. Choices should not be so numerous that the student spends much time trying to determine what choice to accept. A multiple choice or alternate response question that offers several extra items can often be helpful to a student. An alternate-response format that suggests students choose 10 out of 12 test questions for answering or an essay or problem-solving test which advises the students to select 2 out of 3 or 2 out of 4 questions will provide flexibility which can be supportive of the student.

Flexibility also relates to the interpretation of responses of students. Predetermined responses are indicated when the test is developed. However, one must approach the interpretation response with a certain degree of humility. Sometimes the student's knowledge base exceeds the teacher's! Opportunity for the student to support a response is important and should be provided in an examination. A well-developed or theoretically sound response, although not consistent with the pre-determined criteria, should be accepted. The student who knows he/she has a chance brings a more confident manner to the test situation.

Another factor under process and structure is addressed to the timing for providing feedback of results to students, *availability of results*. The feedback principle is seen within the context of diagnostic teaching. It is advisable that results be available to students within a week of testing. The exact timing is often dependent upon the format of the test and the type of test items to be evaluated. Fixed-answer questions, such as multiple choice, alternate response, and others that can be scored easily may be available for feedback more quickly. Free-response questions (essay, problem solving) will necessitate a longer evaluation period, but should still be completed within a week. Final examinations are generally not used for feedback, especially if they are offered during the typical final examination week of a term.

Test Design

An understanding of the process of the development prepares one to consider the actual design of the test. The identification of the objectives to be tested with a clear delineation of the critical elements or test units to be tested requires that the appropriate format for test items be selected.

As mentioned previously, there are two classifications of test items, the fixed-answer question and the free-response question. The decision as to what format to use depends upon the objectives to be evaluated, the purpose of the examination, the number of students to be tested, and the time required for response analysis. A final examination with the demand for immediate feedback, including a compilation of various evaluation strategies for a course grade to be submitted within forty-eight hours, places real constraints on test makers. With small numbers of students, a free-response test may be administered, but with large numbers of students in a limited time frame, the faculty may be forced to rely on fixed-answer items.

The expected behavior is critical in selecting the testing format. The behavior signals the point on the taxonomy that the question must address. Generally, fixed-response questions are limited to the first three cognitive levels (knowledge, comprehension, and application). Free-response questions such as reflective thinking questions are appropriate at most levels beginning with the second one, comprehension. Especially in undergraduate programs the usual test situation does not often go beyond the fourth level, analysis. Affective behaviors may be tested on the first two levels (receiving and responding) by fixed response questions. Free-response questions could be used for the second through fourth level (responding, valuing, and organization of values).

One other factor influencing the selection of test items relates to the intent of the examination—criterion referenced or norm referenced. Norm referenced requires that discriminatory items be incorporated. It is generally expected that a discriminatory item be selected so that the top one-third of the students provide a better response than the lower one-third. It must be remembered, however, that the discriminatory question must be derived from the critical element or test unit. Many test makers use this discriminatory process to provide questions outside the expected content area. A discriminatory question needs to address greater depth of one of the critical elements.

The plan of the test is individual in relation to its purpose and the objectives tested. A one-strategy test may be designed or a multi-strategy test may be the appropriate format. The one-strategy test using fixed-response questions is easily scorable if it is designed so that the format for response is consistent. It is suggested that the easier items appear first so that the testee feels some sense of achievement on the test. It is difficult to state how many items should be included, generally about 115 items of multiple response are achievable in a two-hour examination period. Again, the number is determined by the level of test items; recall items can be answered more quickly than can those demanding higher cognitive skills.

A single-strategy test using free-response questions is often more challenging and demanding of the students. The number of test items varies with the objectives to which test items are addressed. A free response question above the first level can often relate to more than one objective.

A multiple-strategy test enables the test designer to test a wider range of behaviors. A variety also relieves the boredom and tendency to answer questions by guessing as the student reaches the final portion of the examination. Boredom facilitates the onset of fatigue during a test situation.

When multiple strategies are used, it is advisable to section the examination, with each section representing a different strategy. Precise instructions for each section must be provided and the weight of each section should be communicated to the student. Choice in questions within each section to be answered is also helpful to a student.

If the multiple-strategies test includes both types of test items, fixed answer and free response, more time must be provided for the free-response questions. In a situation test, the items may represent both types of questions—again as determined by the behaviors to be tested. Weighing in multi-strategy tests is most important, with the highest weight assigned to the free-response questions unless the latter are only a small part of the test.

Once test items are developed, it is appropriate to test out the items with faculty, colleagues, or other students not involved in the test situation. This experience often helps to identify any ambiguity in the wording or the conveying of a message not compatible with the original intent for the question. The post-test analysis will be discussed subsequently.

Test Question Banks

Computer technology has made preparing tests and revising questions easier for faculty. The process of arranging questions on a test, inserting and deleting questions, and modifying questions based on data obtained from an item analysis is facilitated with computer technology. In addition, a test bank can be developed as a means of classifying and storing test questions in an organized way and then generating tests from the test question bank. Multiple forms of a test can be generated from the same questions. Software packages are available to serve this purpose and, in recent years, some publishers in nursing have provided test banks for faculty use when a particular textbook published by them has been adopted.

With a test bank, test questions are categorized and then stored for future use by faculty. A test bank consists of three data storage systems: a list of subject headings, which are fairly broad to facilitate item retrieval; a situation document containing case studies for use with specific test questions; and test bank document with the test items (Collins et al., 1985). Rizzolo (1985) describes how faculty can create their own test bank using a microcomputer and fairly standard word processing program. Test banks provide faculty with a mechanism for revising items and constructing examinations.

Criteria

In any test development, certain criteria need to be considered in determining its appropriateness for use. Criteria include:

1. Validity — the extent to which the test measures what it is intended to do

2. Reliability — the consistency with which the test measures what it is designed to do

3. Administration — the ease of administration of the test for both faculty and student

4. Cost Effectiveness — the reasonableness of the cost of the test in relation to its development, administration, analysis, and scoring

5. Scorability — the potential for scoring within the confines of time, faculty ability, and fairness

6. Accuracy in preparation of materials

the preparation of the test with regard to clarity of instruction, accuracy of typing, spacing of items, and facility in recording answers

Item Analysis

After administration of a test, faculty should review test questions and identify areas needing revision. Item analysis, which may be hand calculated or computer generated, provides information about individual test questions which then may be used in revising them. Typically, item analysis is done for dichotomously scored items, such as multiple choice and alternate response, although similar procedures have been described for use with essay questions (Layton, 1985).

Item analysis provides three types of information: item difficulty, item discrimination, and the effectiveness of distractors. Item difficulty refers simply to the percentage of students who answered the question correctly. Items that are too difficult can be revised or even discarded from a test, or teaching strategies might be reexamined. Often tests are constructed with items of varying levels of difficulty (Cassidy, 1987). The discrimination index refers to the ability of a particular item to differentiate between learners who achieved higher test scores with those who received lower scores on the test overall. One other component of item analysis involves evaluation of the distractors. Here the teacher can calculate the percentage of students who chose each distractor to provide a measure of which distractors were effective and which were not. Such information provides a basis for revising a distractor. The reader is directed to references in nursing (Cassidy, 1987; Jenkins & Michael, 1986; Layton, 1985) for a discussion of formulas for calculating item difficulty and item discrimination and related examples; other references are included with the recommended readings of this chapter.

Results of an item analysis assist faculty in deciding on possible revisions of a question, whether to retain the item as is, or whether to discard the question. Item analysis does not "tell" the teacher what changes, if any, to make; it provides information about the question on the basis of testee response to contribute to the teacher's decision making.

ETHICAL ISSUES

Any evaluation activity has built into it a moral and ethical component. Educational evaluation is a process of making judgments on the value or worth of an experience, a performance, or a product. The judgments made have implications not only for the present events in the student's life, but they often extend into future events. It is of utmost importance that the qualities of fairness, integrity and justice characterize the value decisions made.

Testing is an evaluation process that is particularly vulnerable to ethical and moral issues because of the perceived power discrepancy between teacher and students which may not be evident in the usual teaching–learning interactions. The means by which the teacher handles this disparity is the critical factor in establishing trust and respect for the worth and dignity of the student.

Thoughtful preparation of the students for the examination, including responding honestly to their concerns, and assurance that test questions are compatible with intended behaviors expressed in the objectives, evidence the teacher's caring about the students and how they perform on the test.

The approach used in correcting the student's paper is an important criterion in judging the teacher's respect for students. The field of knowledge in nursing has so many ambiguities that opportunity for a student to defend a response that is not in accord with the anticipated response of the teacher is essential. When the response is supported by a rational defense, it is the responsibility of the teacher to accept the challenge and alter the grade accordingly. This change is not a matter of willingness on the part of the teacher, but rather it is a requirement in terms of the student's rights.

Teachers convey different messages in testing situations. Although they affirm that testing is designed to determine the quality and perhaps quantity of student knowledge, this intent can be nullified. Actions leading to questioning of the intent include denying student involvement in the testing process except in the testee role, submitting questions that are not congruent with the objectives of the learning experiences, or preparing test items that represent trivia or suggest trickery. There is a danger now that with the increased use of computers for correcting and scoring tests, the teacher will withdraw from the human component of test reading and the process will become dehumanized and routinized.

The management of test results presents another area for consideration relative to student rights. What rights does the student have in the dissemination of a grade obtained on a test? Who has the right to be informed about the grade? What about the practice of posting grades? What rights does the student have when requests for a report of an examination grade are received from a source outside the educational institution? These questions are posed here for consideration of faculty and others relative to student rights and protection of privacy.

SUMMARY

Testing is an integral part of the educational experience, one which can either facilitate or deter the student's learning. Faculty that sincerely answer the three critical questions: Why am I testing? How am I testing? What results am I getting? will design and administer tests that promote the student's desire "to know what I know." Test development is directed by specific purposes and addressed to the essentials. Norm-referenced examinations use a stated norm as a referent while criterion-referenced examinations use an absolute standard as a referent. The latter purpose is most compatible with teacher-developed tests used in a nursing program which stresses competency as the achievement level. All tests must meet criteria of validity, reliability, administerability, cost effectiveness, scorability, and accuracy in preparation of materials.

Because of the significance of testing in our society and the uses of tests in determining directions in life open to individuals, the faculty are held ethically responsible to protect the rights of the testee. Data obtained by results are significant for inclusion in both formative and summative processes in a course. Tests can be purposeful, creative, challenging, interesting, and informative and a valuable component of the learning experiences of students.

REFERENCES

Barnes, R. (1987). Test anxiety in master's students: A comparative study. *Journal of Nursing Education, 26*(1), 12–18.

Benjamin, M., McKeachie, W., Lin, Y. et al. (1981). Test anxiety: Deficits in information processing. *Journal of Educational Psychology, 75*(6), 816–824.

Bigge, M. (1982). *Learning theories for teachers* (4th ed.). New York: Harper & Row.

Bruner, J. (1963). *Process of education*. New York: Vintage Books.

Cassidy, V. R. (1987). Test construction techniques. *Journal of Nursing Staff Development, 3*(4), 154–158.

Collins, M. M., Ellis, A. P., Fiske, J. M., & Genco, H. L. (1985). Computer assisted test bank. *Journal of Nursing Education, 24*(8), 349–350.

Jenkins, H. M., & Michael, M. M. (1986). Using and interpreting item analysis data. *Nurse Educator, 11*(1), 10–14.

Layton, J. M. (1985). Item analysis for teacher-made tests. *Nurse Educator, 10*(4), 27–30.

Lenberg, C. (1979). *The clinical performance examination*. Norwalk, CT: Appleton-Century-Crofts.

Lowman, J. (1984). *Mastering the techniques of teaching*. San Francisco: Jossey-Bass.

Meyers, C. (1986). *Teaching students to think creatively.* San Francisco: Jossey-Bass.

Milton, O., Pollio, H., Eison, J. (1986). *Making sense of college grades.* San Francisco: Jossey-Bass.

Phillips, A. (1988). Reducing nursing students' anxiety level and increasing retention of materials. *Journal of Nursing Education, 27*(1), 35–41.

Rizzolo, M. A. (1987). Guidelines for creating test question banks. *Computers in Nursing, 5*(2), 65–69.

RECOMMENDED READINGS

Benner, P. (1982). Issues in competency based testing. *Nursing Outlook, 30,* 303–309.

Beyer, F. (1984). The comprehensive nursing achievement test as predictor of performance on the NCLEX-RN. *Nursing & Health Care, 5,* 191–195.

Bloom, B., Hastings, J., & Madaus, G. (1971). *Handbook on formative and summative evaluation of student learning.* New York: McGraw-Hill.

Bloom, B. (Ed.) (1966). *Taxonomy of educational objectives: Book I, Cognitive domain.* New York: Longman.

Cassidy, V. R. (1987). Response changing and student achievement on objective tests. *Journal of Nursing Education, 26*(2), 60–62.

Chickering, A. (1983). Grades: One more tilt at the windmill. *AAHE Bulletin, 35*(8), 10–13.

Ebel, R. L., & Frisbie, D. A. (1986). *Essentials of educational measurement* (4th ed.). Englewood Cliffs, NJ: Prentice-Hall.

Eison, J. (1981). A new instrument for assessing student orientation toward grades and learning. *Psychological Reports, 38,* 917–924.

Feletti, G., Neame, R. (1981). Curricular strategies for reducing examination anxiety. *Higher Education, 10*(6), 675–686.

Flynn, M. K., & Reese, J. L. (1988). Development and evaluation of classroom tests: A practical application. *Journal of Nursing Education, 27*(2), 61–65.

Fredrickson, N. (1984). The real test bias: Influences in testing and learning. *American Psychologist, 39*(3), 193–202.

Gordy, H. (1984). Crisis aspect of test taking: How the teachers can help. *Nursing & Health Care, 5*(2), 100–105.

Gronlund, N. E., & Linn, R. L. (1990). *Measurement and evaluation in teaching* (6th ed.). New York: Macmillan.

Hopkins, C. D., & Antes, R. L. (1985). *Classroom measurement and evaluation* (2nd ed.). Itasca, IL: F.E. Peacock.

Hopkins, K. D., Stanley, J. C., & Hopkins, B. R. (1990). *Educational and psychological measurement and evaluation* (7th ed.). Englewood Cliffs, NJ: Prentice-Hall.

Howard, E. P. (1985). Applying the Rasch model to test administration. *Journal of Nursing Education, 24*(8), 340–343.

Livingston, S. A., & Zieky, M. J. (1982). *Passing scores: A manual for setting standards on educational and occupational tests.* Princeton, NJ: Princeton Educational Testing Service.

McFarland, M. (1983). Contract grading in nursing education. *Nursing Educator, 8*(4), 3–6.

Menacher, J., & Morris, V. (1985). Testing, civil rights and the courts. *Educational Forum, 49*(3), 285–296.

Mentzer, T. (1982). Response bias in multiple choice tests. *Educational & Psychological Measurement, 42,* 437–444.

Nichols, E. G., & Miller, G. K. (1984). Interreader agreement on comprehensive essay examinations. *Journal of Nursing Education, 23*(2), 64–69.

Ross, G., & Ross, M. (1977). Using the computer to prepare multiple choice examinations. *Journal of Nursing Education, 16,* 32.

Schneider, H. (1984). *Effective test construction in the health professions.* Jackson, MS: H. and B. Co.

Stedman, C. (1985). Testing for competence: Lessons from health professions. *Educational Forum, 49*(2), 199–210.

Vallerand, A. H. (1988). Differences in test performance and learner satisfaction among nurses with varying autonomy levels. *Journal of Continuing Education in Nursing, 19*(5), 92–98.

Van Ort, S., & Cardea, J. (1986). Test-taking workshops for nursing students. *Nurse Educator, 11*(3), 38–40.

Van Ort, S., & Hazzard, M. E. (1985). A guide for evaluation of test items. *Nurse Educator, 10*(5), 13–15.

10

Preparation of Tests Within Nursing Process Framework

Testing practices within the framework of the nursing process are an important component of the system of evaluation in a nursing program. Testing of the cognitive or theoretical component of the nursing process provides data on the student's knowledge of the process and ability to use it in simulated situations. As students progress through the nursing program, experiences provide for use of the nursing process with increasingly more complex problems. Development of test questions which reflect application of theory and analytical thinking should be included in the system of evaluation. Multiple-choice testing within the framework of the nursing process model also provides essential experience for students in answering questions similar to those found on the licensing examination.

NURSING PROCESS

In clinical practice the nurse uses his or her abilities to meet the health needs of clients, individuals, families, and other groups, in a range of settings. Clinical practice is a dynamic comprised of cognitive, psychomotor, and affective behaviors synthesized into the framework of the nursing process.

The nursing process is the methodology of nursing practice, a problem-solving method consisting of a series of nursing actions directed toward the goal of promoting an optimal level of client health. These actions or operations are goal directed, interrelated, and dynamic. They include:

1. Intellectual operations, such as critical thinking, problem solving, decision making, and application of a synthesis of concepts, theories, and ideas.

2. Value judgments based on respect for the dignity and worth of the client.

3. Psychomotor skills used in both assessment and intervention.

The nursing literature contains many references about the nursing process and its use in practice with different types of clients. The intent here is not to review these references but to examine the nursing process in terms of behaviors to be achieved by students that are amenable to evaluation. These behaviors are a major component of clinical evaluation and are examined within this framework in the next chapter. In addition to evaluating students' use of nursing process behaviors in the clinical field, knowledge of the steps of the process and ability to apply this knowledge and associated skills to a client situation may be evaluated through paper-and-pencil testing and other evaluation strategies such as media, simulations, and problem-solving items.

The nursing process is described generally as consisting of four or five steps. While some experts describe four steps: assessment, plan, implementation, and evaluation (Reilly & Oermann, 1985; Yura & Walsh, 1988), others identify five or more: assessment, diagnosis, plan, implementation, and evaluation (Alfaro, 1986; Gordon, 1987; Ziegler, Vaughan-Wrobel, & Erlen, 1986). In conceptualizing the nursing process with four steps, diagnosis is considered as the final component of assessment; with five or more steps, nursing diagnosis becomes a separate phase. Although sometimes viewed in the literature as a linear process, the phases of the nursing process are interrelated and not always carried out in a step-by-step fashion. In assessment, for example, data are collected to arrive at a nursing diagnosis which in turn provides the basis for the plan, interventions, and evaluation. Assessment, however, also takes place during these other steps of the nursing process. Additional data may be collected after the plan is established and implemented because of continuing health problems of the client.

The nursing process is primarily cognitive requiring skill in clinical judgment. The formation of clinical judgments by nurses, decisions as to observations to make in clinical situations, nursing diagnoses, and related actions, is embodied in the nursing process (Miller & Malcolm, 1990). The nursing process was once viewed as simple problem solving but is now known to involve more complex thinking. In addition to cognitive skills, the nursing process also requires psychomotor skills in the collection of data and nursing interventions. The nurse's values are reflected in the nursing process through the nurse's interactional skills including use of touch and nonverbal and verbal communication, types of data obtained and then interpreted, and decisions made regarding care. Value judgments based on respect for the inherent worth and dignity of the client are inherent in all steps of the nursing process.

In assisting students in the development of skills associated with the nursing process, and in their evaluation, the teacher is concerned with behaviors drawn from the three domains of learning—cognitive, psychomotor, and affective—integrated in practice. The behaviors inherent in the nursing process may be incorporated in the objectives for learning and used as a basis for evaluation. Evaluation strategies can then be developed to assess competency in using the nursing process in a variety of settings and clinical situations.

Although classification of steps of the nursing process varies with the particular author, in general the following four steps are identified:

1. Assessment
2. Planning
3. Implementation
4. Evaluation

The following behaviors are suggested for each step of the nursing process.

Assessment

1. Recognizes possible health problems, providing direction to the collection of data.
2. Makes relevant observations.
3. Conducts purposeful interviews.
4. Uses appropriate resources for data gathering.
5. Uses technical data gathering skills when relevant.
6. Identifies cues in the data.
7. Collects data regarding goals of care and plans of other health care professionals.
8. Relates client's and family's responses to health and illness to their sociocultural background.

9. Accepts the rights of clients to their own philosophy, moral code, and life style.
10. Seeks to avoid interference of own biases in the collection and interpretation of data.
11. Identifies client's responses that can be used in meeting health needs.
12. Interprets data in terms of nursing models, relevant concepts and theories from other fields, and research.
13. Identifies significant relationships among the data.
14. Generates tentative diagnostic hypotheses.
15. Gathers additional data to support or reject the hypotheses.
16. Differentiates between own data analysis and that identified for a typical situation.
17. Establishes a nursing diagnosis(es) from the hypotheses.
18. Establishes a priority of needs.

Planning

1. Involves the client and family in determining short- and long-term goals.
2. Develops goals for nursing care based on nursing diagnoses.
3. Involves the client and family in development of the plan of care.
4. Selects nursing measures determined to be most effective in meeting goals of care.
5. Establishes a nursing care plan consistent with the goals.
6. Communicates plan of care to other nursing personnel.
7. Relates plan of care to those of other disciplines.

Implementation

1. Carries out nursing measures consistent with scientific concepts.
2. Uses technical skills competently.
3. Maintains a therapeutic environment.
4. Informs client of actions inherent in the plan of care.
5. Uses appropriate channels for communicating information to others.

6. Records significant information accurately.

7. Protects client's legal rights and rights to privacy and confidentiality.

8. Encourages client to use own capabilities to maximum potential.

9. Assists client and family to accept realistic limitations imposed by health problem.

10. Accepts responsibility to act on behalf of the client when conflict exists between the nurse's and client's moral and ethical code.

11. Applies appropriate measures to cope with barriers to effective communication.

12. Initiates referrals based on identified needs to selected community resources.

13. Teaches the client and family in relation to identified learning needs.

14. Works with clients and others to provide for continuity of care.

Evaluation

1. Uses criteria to measure the effectiveness of nursing interventions in terms of goals.

2. Uses evaluation data to assess the process of nursing care from the perspective of each step and its interrelationship.

3. Revises plan as indicated in the evaluation.

These behaviors may be modified for particular courses and clinical experiences to reflect the emphasis of the experience and subsequent evaluation. Specific areas of data gathering for the maternity client, for instance, may be reflected in the objectives designated for assessment. The behaviors suggested here provide a framework for faculty as they develop nursing process objectives for their program and individual courses within it, depending on the particular course as well as the teacher's own perspective of the nursing process.

Evaluation of Nursing Process Behaviors

In evaluating student's competency in using the nursing process, most of the data are collected typically in the clinical field as the learner interacts with and provides care to the client. In the clinical field, the teacher has an opportunity to observe the student's *use* of the process with clients with varied health problems and evaluate related competencies through different clinical evaluation strategies. There is also a need, however, for evaluation of the theoretical elements in the nursing process prior to its use in practice. Evaluation of nursing process behaviors outside of the clinical field, through different strategies in the classroom and learning laboratory, provides an indication of the student's knowledge of the nursing process, its dynamic, and the ability to use it in simulated situations. This evaluation may be through paper-and-pencil testing, with multiple choice, multiple response, and essay items being particularly relevant; problem-solving strategies; videotaping and other media; and different types of simulations.

Current practice suggests that in paper-and-pencil testing in nursing, questions often focus on scientific rationale and principles related to practice and the selection of interventions to use with a particular client problem. Fewer test questions are written on data to collect in a clinical situation, the analysis of data to derive a nursing diagnosis, setting goals for care, evaluation of the effectiveness of an intervention, delivery of care, and progress of the client in meeting health goals. Test questions developed within the framework of the nursing process provide data on the student's skill in assessment, planning, selection of interventions, and evaluation, for both formative and summative purposes.

Such testing practices are an important component of the system of evaluation in a nursing program. Nursing process testing can occur throughout the curriculum relative to the theoretical component of each clinical nursing course. As the student progresses through the program, experiences provide for use of the nursing process with increasingly complex nursing problems requiring greater analysis. Questions that require analytical problem-solving ability can be included in test situations so that the student's process of logical and rational thinking can be evidenced. This is particularly relevant for students in the upper levels of a nursing program.

Nursing process testing also provides experience for students in the nursing program to engage in testing similar to the model used in The National Council Licensure Examination for Registered Nurses (NCLEX-RN) so they are familiar with this type of test. The NCLEX-RN is based on the nursing process with a multiple-choice question format. Although research is not yet available as to the relationship of nursing process testing within an educational program and achievement on the NCLEX-RN, studies have found a correlation between success on the NCLEX-RN and completion of Mosby *AssessTest* (Hughes & Ping, 1987; Jenks et al., 1989; McKinney et al., 1988). Mosby *AssessTest*, and other similar standardized examinations such as the National League for Nursing (NLN) Diagnostic Readiness Test for RN Licensure, provide feedback as to areas in which review is needed as well as give practice in answering questions based on the nursing process. Baradell et al. (1990) recommend practice in taking tests organized around the components of the NCLEX-RN. Integration of test questions based on the nursing process throughout the program assists in identifying areas in which further learning is needed and practice in answering questions on each step of the process.

NCLEX-RN

Professions by their nature serve society through their specialized knowledge and skills and, as such, are obligated to ensure safety in practice and a particular level of competence of its practitioners. Licensure examinations are one way of assuring a safe level of practice among professionals. Early in the history of licensure in nursing, each state wrote its own rules and regulations and developed its own licensure examination. In 1944, the NLN assumed responsibility for the examination, and by 1952 all states were using the same test, although each with its own passing score (Matassarin-Jacobs, 1989). Responsibility for the examination was assumed later by the American Nurses' Association, then the National Council of State Boards of Nursing (NCSBN). In 1982, significant changes were made by the NCSBN in the examination. Scoring changed from a normative-referenced to criterion-referenced system. Matassarin-Jacobs (1989) believes the move to criterion-referencing was positive, ensuring that minimal standards associated with entry level practice are met. The other significant change in the examination in 1982 was the development of questions based on the nursing process, reflecting an integrated view of nursing rather than testing specific subject areas. The NCLEX-RN was revised again in 1988 based on a job analysis study (Kane et al., 1986). As of 1988, no scores are reported for the examination, only pass–fail.

The test plan for the NCLEX-RN addresses two components: phases of the nursing process and needs of clients with commonly occurring health problems. The phases of the nursing process measured in the examination include assessment, analysis, planning, implementation, and evaluation. The health needs of clients are categorized in four areas: (a) safe, effective environment; (b) physiological integrity; (c) psychosocial integrity; and (d) health promotion/maintenance (NCSBN, 1987a). The examination includes test questions developed at the knowledge, comprehension, application, and analysis levels of the taxonomy of the cognitive domain. While the number of items developed at each taxonomic level is not specified, most questions are at the application and analysis levels (NCSBN, 1987a, p. 1).

Research is ongoing to determine the feasibility of using a Computerized Adaptive Test (CAT) mode for administering the NCLEX-RN. With CAT, each candidate's test is assembled interactively as the individual is being tested.

With each question answered by the candidate, the computer calculates a competence estimate based on earlier answers, scans available test questions, and selects the best one for the candidate (NCSBN, 1989). Other advantages of CAT are that candidates will be able to schedule the examination at their convenience, near the time when they graduate; the examination will be self-paced, better reflecting individual variations among candidates; and the results will be available to candidates immediately upon conclusion of the examining session (NCSBN, 1987b).

Research to examine the feasibility of incorporating computerized clinical simulations into the NCLEX-RN is underway. Computerized Simulation Testing (CST) presents a series of clinical simulations to which the candidate responds. The condition of the client and problems presented vary based on the health problem being tested and the candidate's own responses. The candidate is able, any time throughout the simulation, to collect data, review the client's record, and perform nursing interventions in any sequence (NCSBN, 1990). The interventions, which are uncued and specified by free keyboard entry, include a full range of nursing care measures (Bersky, 1990). It has been suggested that CST offers an improved method of assessing problem-solving and decision-making abilities of the candidate. In addition to the possible use of computerized simulations as part of the licensure examination, some professionals believe that observing actual performance in real or simulated situations is also important in this process (Stedman, 1985).

Research to identify predictors of success on the NCLEX-RN is limited although increasing within recent years. McKinney et al. (1988) found significant positive correlations between cumulative grade point average (GPA); Mosby *AssessTest*; preentrance test scores (i.e., SAT); prenursing, nursing theory, and clinical GPA; and performance on the NCLEX-RN. Age, gender, and Type A personality were not predictors. When multiple regression was used, preentrance test scores, GPA, Mosby *AssessTest* scores, and courses repeated were significant predictors of success on the NCLEX-RN. Performance in prenursing courses has been identified as an important predictor of success on the NCLEX-RN (Glick et al., 1986; Payne & Duffy, 1986; Quick et al., 1985). Findings also suggest that grades in specific nursing courses and cumulative GPA at graduation are other predictors (Glick et al., 1986; Krupa et al., 1988; Lengacher & Keller, 1990; McKinney et al., 1988; Payne & Duffy, 1986). Jenks et al. (1989) found a strong correlation between success on the NCLEX-RN and the theory component of clinical nursing courses similar to other studies (Glick et al., 1986; Payne & Duffy, 1986). Although additional research in this area is needed, it has been suggested that students whose academic patterns suggest possible difficulty in passing the NCLEX-RN can be identified early in the nursing program and instructional strategies be implemented for these learners.

Development of Multiple-Choice Test

In developing questions within the framework of the nursing process, the teacher begins with specifying the total number of items to be included and then the items to be developed for each step of the process in terms of the stated objectives of the course. With some tests greater emphasis may be given to evaluation of one particular area of the process, for instance, assessment, depending on the weight given to those objectives in the instruction and focus of the examination. Mapping out the total test and the number of questions to be developed for each step of the process enables faculty to balance test questions and ensure representation of the objectives. Another important decision at this point relates to the types of test questions to be used, for instance, multiple recognition, essay, problem solving, and others, in the evaluation. While the NCLEX-RN uses multiple-choice for testing, other types of test items and evaluation strategies might also be incorporated into the testing situation.

In any test the teacher may write individual discrete items on each step of the nursing process or may develop questions around a client or other clinical situation. In using client situations for nursing process testing, the situation provides the context for problem solving and specific data relevant to the questions which are asked. With this format questions have a relationship to one another and to the clinical situation described in the test, similar to the NCLEX-RN. When using clinical situations as the framework for writing nursing process questions, data may be added to the situation to expand it and more effectively lead into other questions. Only relevant data, however, should be included as extraneous material may distract the student as well as increase reading time unless the intent of the objective being evaluated relates to analysis of data.

Test questions developed around clinical situations require preplanning to identify significant data to be included in the situation and whether or not new information will be added to it at some other point in testing. The order in which questions are asked does not necessarily reflect the sequence of steps of the nursing process but instead varies with how the situation is developed. Schneider (1984) recommends limiting questions related to one particular client situation as students may forget important data as they proceed through the questions.

Objectives on the nursing process may be written at the knowledge, comprehension, application, and analysis levels depending on the course and level of the learner. Test questions, therefore, also may be developed at these different cognitive levels, similar to the NCLEX-RN. Questions at the knowledge level reflect recall of specific facts, principles, and other information related to each step of the nursing process. At the comprehension level, items are designed to measure student understanding of these concepts and ability to explain and describe them. It is at the application level where test questions need to measure *use* of knowledge, that is, application of concepts, principles, and theories, in assessment, planning, implementation, and evaluation. Bloom (1956) indicates that test questions at this level examine application of knowledge in a particular situation. Development of multiple-choice questions at the analysis level, however, is more difficult. Such items require students to analyze the client situation and other information presented to identify critical elements within it and relationships among them, that is, derive meaning from the situation using resources outside of the data at hand. Bloom suggests that testing ability to analyze is carried out most effectively when the material to be analyzed is new to the student and appropriate questions are then asked about it. In this way the test questions are more likely to examine analytical abilities since the student does not have an opportunity to simply recall an analysis from previous discussion of a similar situation. In developing questions at the analysis level for the nursing process, then, the teacher is concerned with presenting material new to the learner which requires analytical thinking in order to respond to the related questions.

Preparation and use of various test formats have been discussed earlier. This chapter addresses the preparation of multiple-choice items for four levels of the cognitive taxonomy in terms of the steps of the nursing process. Illustrations of test items developed at the knowledge level of the taxonomy are included here but generally should not appear in a test related to clinical nursing practice where handling of information, not recall, is essential. The authors have reservations about multiple-choice questions being used to test the critical thinking activity entailed in the analysis level of the taxonomy. Examples are offered here for consideration by the reader.

Test Questions: Assessment

Test questions evaluating student competency in assessment include items on subjective and objective data to be gathered relative to the client, verifying and communicating data, and analyzing data to identify health care problems and establish nursing diagnoses. While the specific test question relates to the objective being evaluated, the following examples of stems may be used in the development of questions on assessment.

Data Collection

1. In the assessment, the nurse should collect which of the following data?
2. Which of the following information should be collected as a priority in the assessment process?
3. Which one of the following questions should be asked by the nurse in the assessment of the client/family?
4. What additional data need to be collected to establish the nursing diagnoses?
5. Because of . . . , which one of the following areas of data collection is most significant?
6. Which of the following resources should be used in gathering data?

Data Analysis

1. These data support the nursing diagnosis of _____.
2. Which of the following nursing diagnoses is appropriate for this client?
3. The client's health care problems include _____.
4. Which one of the following needs is of greatest priority at this time?

These examples of stems are by no means exhaustive but are intended instead to illustrate how they may be written to examine knowledge of the assessment process and its application in the testing situation.

Questions on assessment at different cognitive levels are illustrated below. Because assessment includes both the collection and analysis of data, additional illustrations are included to give the reader a perspective of the type of item that may be developed for this step of the nursing process. In the examples which follow for assessment, and the other phases of the nursing process, only multiple-choice questions are included since this is the format of testing in the NCLEX-RN.

BEHAVIORAL OBJECTIVE	TEST ITEM
C1.12 Identifies characteristics of different types of tumors.	Which one of the following characteristics which the patient reported is most likely to suggest a benign tumor? 1. One single lump 2. Fully movable 3. Irregular, solid, hard 4. Nontender, painless

BEHAVIORAL OBJECTIVE	TEST ITEM

BEHAVIORAL OBJECTIVE

C2.2   Describes areas of data collection for a patient receiving oxygen therapy.

TEST ITEM

Which one of the following sources of information is *least* significant in assessment of the client receiving oxygen?
1. Orientation to time and place
2. Level of consciousness
3. Change in motor ability
4. Cognitive functioning

C2.2   Describes characteristics of different breathing patterns.

Hyperventilation is characterized by
1. increased respiration rate.
2. decreased depth in respiration.
3. irregular breathing.
4. labored breathing with increased rate.

C3.0   Identifies data to be collected for care of clients with closed head injury.

Mr. Smith is admitted to the emergency room with a severe headache and weakness of the right leg one month following a closed head injury. Mr. Smith is drowsy and irritable. His vital signs are: BP 166/100, P 68, R 16, and T 99. Which one of the following areas of data collection would be the best indicator of Mr. Smith's neurological status?
1. Vital signs
2. Pupillary response
3. Motor ability
4. State of consciousness

C3.0   Identifies nursing diagnoses for clients with neurological problems.

Which one of the following nursing diagnoses is of the greatest priority at this time for Mr. Smith?
1. Sleep pattern disturbance
2. Impaired physical mobility
3. Pain
4. Altered thought processes

C3.0   Uses communication theory in examining interaction patterns of family members.

Which one of the following combinations of behavioral responses suggests a placating mode of interaction?

BEHAVIORAL OBJECTIVE	TEST ITEM
	1. Ingratiating with frequent descriptions of others as "sweet," "so nice," "such a lovely person."
	2. Always trying to please and be liked; avoids confrontation at all costs.
	3. Trailing off in mid-sentences; uses stories, words, and tangents which lack relevance.
	4. Stays only with the facts; is reasonable; avoids feelings.
C4.2 Analyzes needs of clients with chronic respiratory problems.	A patient with moderately advanced emphysema was preparing for discharge the following day to his apartment where he lives alone. During the evening, he summoned the nurse with frantic ringing of the bell. When the nurse entered the room, she saw the patient diaphoresing, trembling, and evidencing signs of anxiety. Which one of the following reasons reflects a major concern of patients with emphysema?
	1. The patient fears that once he is home, no one will be available in the event of a respiratory crisis.
	2. The patient is experiencing separation anxiety.
	3. The patient is apprehensive about resuming his self care.
	4. The patient fears he will experience another respiratory crisis which will delay his discharge.

Test Questions: Planning

Test questions on the planning process focus on setting goals, both short- and long-term, for meeting client needs; selecting nursing measures for achieving these goals; and developing care plans with input from patient and family and collaboration with other health care professionals involved in the care and its delivery. Examples of stems appropriate particularly for questions on planning care include:

1. The goal of care for this client is ———.
2. Which one of the following goals is of greatest priority?
3. Which one of these nursing measures should be included in the plan of care?
4. To meet the goal of . . . , which nursing intervention(s) would be most appropriate to include in the plan of care?
5. Which one of these resources should be incorporated in the plan of care?
6. Which one of the following statements is most appropriate for inclusion in the written nursing care plan?

BEHAVIORAL OBJECTIVE	TEST ITEM
C1.12 Identifies appropriate nursing measures for clients with dentures.	Which one of the following actions is appropriate for a patient with dentures? 1. Floss to remove stains between teeth. 2. Wrap in wash cloth to prevent breakage. 3. Soak in mouthwash to remove plaque. 4. Store in labeled container when not in mouth.
C2.2 Describes goals for clients in respiratory distress.	A priority goal for a patient admitted in acute respiratory distress is to 1. decrease the patient's anxiety and resulting respiratory distress. 2. prepare the patient and family for the stress associated with acute care. 3. obtain critical data for establishing the diagnoses. 4. maintain an airway to ensure respiratory functioning.

BEHAVIORAL OBJECTIVE	TEST ITEM
C3.0 Develops plans for care of clients with casts, in traction, and with other related devices.	Michael, a 4-year-old with a fractured femur, is discharged with a cast on his right leg. The cast is still damp. Which one of the following actions should be included in the teaching plan for the mother? 1. Dry the cast with a hair dryer. 2. Elevate the leg on pillows. 3. Cover the cast with plastic until dry. 4. Grasp the cast firmly with fingers when moving the leg.
C4.1 Identifies nursing actions for inclusion in the plan of care.	Ms. S., a 40-year-old professional, is admitted to the psychiatric unit. On admission she tells the nurse that "life is hopeless." Since her admission, she is seen pacing the halls and wringing her hands almost continuously. Which one of these nursing actions is most appropriate at this time for inclusion in her care plan? 1. Accept her behavior as a part of her illness requiring no further intervention. 2. Introduce yourself to her with a positive approach and smile. 3. Walk with her stating an understanding of her feelings. 4. Reassure her that life and her own situation will get better.

Test Questions: Implementation

Evaluation of the student's understanding of the implementation phase of the nursing process relates to the learner's knowledge of principles underlying nursing actions, for specific client problems and to meet established goals, and the relationship between the assessment and nursing actions. Test questions for this step of the nursing process include knowledge of nursing measures to be implemented and their underlying scientific base, principles of organizing care, specific measures to promote optimal client functioning, strategies for teaching and counseling clients and families, and documentation of the care provided and its results. Stems useful in writing implementation questions, although similar to some of those identified with planning, emphasize the completion of nursing actions and performance of interventions. Selected illustrations follow:

1. The nursing actions should be performed in the following sequence:
2. Which one of the following nursing interventions should be implemented immediately?
3. The patient should be referred to which of the following resources?
4. Following this diagnostic test/surgery/procedure/intervention, which nursing measure(s) should be implemented?
5. Which one of these nursing measures is essential?
6. Which one of these statements by the nurse is appropriate?
7. Which one of these explanations/instructions should be given to the client/family?
8. Which one of the statements that follow would most accurately communicate to other nurses and health team members the client's response?

BEHAVIORAL OBJECTIVE

C1.12   Identifies treatment for magnesium sulfate toxicity.

TEST ITEM

The antidote for magnesium sulfate toxicity for a patient with a hypertension of pregnancy is
1. lidocaine.
2. narcan.
3. calcium gluconate.
4. sodium bicarbonate.

C2.2   Describes selected therapeutic diets.

You are teaching Mr. S. about a low sodium diet which he is to follow. He tells you the foods he eats typically for lunch. Which one of these foods is acceptable?
1. Corn beef on rye
2. Soup prepared from packages
3. Beer
4. Baked chicken legs

BEHAVIORAL OBJECTIVE	TEST ITEM

C3.0 Selects responses appropriate for therapeutic communication.

Mrs. A. tells the nurse that she is scared to death that her son is taking drugs. Which one of the following statements would be a therapeutic response?
1. "Let's talk about your being scared to death."
2. "Tomorrow I will bring some pamphlets on substance abuse for you."
3. "We have an excellent clinic that helps persons abusing drugs."
4. "Perhaps your fear is not based on facts."

C4.2 Analyzes nursing actions and their outcomes on the basis of scientific rationale.

A patient, three days after surgery, was experiencing difficulty in sleeping because of low grade pain and discomfort. The nurse rubbed the patient's back and changed her position to relieve stress on the operative site. According to gate control theory, which one of the following therapeutic actions brought relief from the discomfort?
1. Decreased the patient's perception of pain thus altering the interpretation of pain stimulus.
2. Stimulated small fibers to increase the inhibition of large afferent nerve vessels which conduct pain impulse.
3. Stimulated large afferent nerve vessels to increase the inhibition of small fibers which conduct pain impulse.
4. Provided distraction to the afferent nerve vessels.

Test Questions: Evaluation

The last step of the nursing process, evaluation, is concerned with the quality dimension of care. Questions developed to assess student knowledge and skill in evaluation may focus on the extent to which goals of care and client outcomes were achieved, the process used in care of the client, and events in the clinical setting which may have influenced care. Test items on ways in which a care plan might be revised, reflecting evaluation data, may also be developed. Stems useful in developing test questions on evaluation include:

1. Which one of these client responses indicates the nursing interventions are effective?
2. Which one of the following responses indicates that the medication/ treatment/intervention is achieving the desired effect?
3. Based on these observations, which one of the following goals has been/not been achieved?
4. Which behavior/response/observation indicates improvement in the client's condition?
5. Which one of these statements by the client/family indicates an understanding of the health problem/instructions/diet/etc.?
6. The following revision is indicated in the plan of care based on these client responses:
7. The client should be observed for which of the following side effects?

BEHAVIORAL OBJECTIVE	TEST ITEM
C1.12 Lists side effects of selected medications.	Which one of the following symptoms indicates a side effect of dilantin? 1. Hypertension 2. Skin rash 3. Urinary retention 4. Hypoglycemia
C2.2 Describes client responses indicating effectiveness of selected medications.	Which one of the following client responses is *not* significant in indicating drug effectiveness during digitalization? 1. Improved pulse rate and rhythm 2. Restlessness 3. Relief of dyspnea 4. Increased tolerance to mild exercise

BEHAVIORAL OBJECTIVE	TEST ITEM
C3.0 Assesses client understanding following instruction.	Ms. C. is taught how to use the Triflow. Which one of these actions which she demonstrated indicates she needs more teaching? 1. able to raise 2 of 3 balls. 2. blows into the mouthpiece. 3. splints her incision. 4. asks for pain medication.
C4.2 Relates client behavior to evaluation of self care status.	In evaluating changes in a patient's behavior toward self-care, all but one of the following questions are relevant. Which one of these questions is *not* pertinent? 1. How has the patient adjusted to the routine of the unit? 2. Does the patient's behavior reflect an appropriate level of independence? 3. Has the patient's knowledge of health status developed sufficiently? 4. What new skills and capacities have the patient and family developed?

Test questions developed within the framework of the nursing process enable the teacher to evaluate student understanding and competency in use of the nursing process in terms of paper-and-pencil testing and provide for students practice in answering questions similar to those included in the NCLEX-RN. In many instances these questions will be developed around a clinical situation with the situation providing the data needed to evaluate application of the nursing process. In other tests, individual questions on the different steps of the process may be more appropriate depending on the objectives to be evaluated.

SUMMARY

Testing of the cognitive or theoretical component of the nursing process provides data on the student's knowledge of the process and ability to use it in simulated situations. As students progress through the nursing program, experiences provide for use of the nursing process with increasingly more complex problems. Development of test questions within the framework of the nursing process provides data on the student's understanding of assessment, planning, implementation, and evaluation for specific client problems. This evaluation is useful for both formative and summative purposes. Over a period of time, student development of competency, and need for further instruction, in the nursing process becomes evident. Multiple-choice testing within the framework of the nursing process model also provides essential experience for students in answering questions similar to those found on the licensing examination.

In developing questions within the framework of the nursing process, test items may be written on data to collect in a clinical situation, the analysis of data to derive a nursing diagnosis, setting goals for care, developing plans of care, selecting appropriate nursing measures, and evaluating the effectiveness of an intervention and delivery of care and progress of the client in meeting health goals. The teacher begins by identifying the objectives to be evaluated and specifying the number of items to be written. Multiple-choice questions may be written for all phases of the nursing process at the first four levels of the cognitive taxonomy: knowledge, comprehension, application, and analysis. The authors question the validity of test items written at the analytic level in multiple-choice format, because of the critical thinking skills required. Testing for cognitive competency within the framework of the nursing process represents an important evaluation strategy for faculty, particularly in clinical nursing courses where use of information is paramount.

REFERENCES

Alfaro, R. (1986). *Application of nursing process.* Philadelphia: J. B. Lippincott.

Baradell, J. G., Durham, C. F., Angel. B. F., Kaufman, J. S., & Lowdermilk, D. (1990). A comprehensive approach to preparation for NCLEX-RN. *Journal of Nursing Education, 29*(3), 109–113.

Bersky, A. (1990, May). Personal communication.

Bloom, B. S. (1956). *Taxonomy of educational objectives. Handbook I: Cognitive domain.* New York: David McKay.

Glick, O. J., McClelland, E., & Yang, J. C. (1986). NCLEX-RN: Predicting the performance of graduates of an integrated baccalaureate nursing program. *Journal of Professional Nursing, 2*(2), 98–103.

Gordon, M. (1987). *Nursing diagnosis: Process and application* (2nd ed.). New York: McGraw-Hill.

Hughes, P., & Ping, J. (1987). *The Mosby ASSESSTEST as a predictor of performance on the NCLEX-RN.* Princeton, NJ: Educational Testing Service.

Jenks, J., Selekman, J., Bross, T., & Paquet, M. (1989). Success in NCLEX-RN: Identifying predictors and optional timing for intervention. *Journal of Nursing Education, 28*(3), 112–118.

Kane, M., Kingsbury, C., Colton, D., & Estes, C. (1986). *A study of nursing practice and role delineation, and job analysis of entry-level performance of registered nurses.* Chicago: National Council of State Boards of Nursing.

Krupa, K. C., Quick, M. M., & Whitley, T. W. (1988). The effectiveness of nursing grades in predicting performance on the NCLEX-RN. *Journal of Professional Nursing, 4*(4), 294–298.

Lengacher, C. A., & Keller, R. (1990). Academic predictors of success on the NCLEX-RN examination for associate degree nursing students. *Journal of Nursing Education, 29*(4), 163–169.

Matassarin-Jacobs, E. (1989). The nursing licensure process and the NCLEX-RN. *Nurse Educator, 14*(6), 32–35.

McKinney, J., Small, S., O'Dell, N., & Coonrod, B. A. (1988). Identification of predictors of success for the NCLEX and students at risk for NCLEX failure in a baccalaureate nursing program. *Journal of Professional Nursing, 4*(1), 55–59.

Miller, M. A., & Malcolm, N. A. (1990). Critical thinking in the nursing curriculum. *Nursing & Health Care, 11*(2), 67–73.

National Council of State Boards of Nursing. (1987a). *NCLEX-RN: Test plan for the National Council Licensure Examination for Registered Nurses.* Chicago: Author.

National Council of State Boards of Nursing. (1987b). Research continues: Computer adaptive testing update. *Issues, 8*(5), 3, 6–8.

National Council of State Boards of Nursing. (1989, September 26). News: Eight states selected as field test sites for NCLEX-RN computerized adaptive testing. Chicago: Author.

National Council of State Boards of Nursing. (1990, April). Fact sheet: CST: Computerized clinical simulation testing project. Chicago: Author

Quick, M., Krupa, K., & Whitley, T. (1985). Using admission data to predict success on the NCLEX-RN in a baccalaureate program. *Journal of Professional Nursing, 1,* 364–368.

Payne, M., & Duffy, M. (1986). An investigation of predictability of NCLEX-RN scores of BSN graduates using academic predictors. *Journal of Professional Nursing, 2*(5), 326–332.

Reilly, D. E., & Oermann, M. H. (1985). *The clinical field: Its use in nursing education.* Norwalk, CT: Appleton-Century-Crofts.

Schneider, H. (1984). *Effective test construction in the health professions.* Jackson, MS: H. and B. Hess Co.

Stedman, C. H. (1985). Testing for competence: Lessons from health professions. *The Educational Forum, 49*(2), 199–210.

Yura, H., & Walsh, M. B. (1988). *The nursing process* (5th ed.). Norwalk, Ct: Appleton & Lange.

Ziegler, S. M., Vaughan-Wrobel, B. C., & Erlen, J. A. (1986). *Nursing process, nursing diagnosis, nursing knowledge.* Norwalk, CT: Appleton-Century-Crofts.

RECOMMENDED READINGS

American Nurses' Association. (1973). *Standards: Nursing practice.* Kansas City, MO: Author.

Benner, P. (1984). *From novice to expert: Excellence and power in clinical nursing practice.* Menlo Park, CA: Addison-Wesley.

Benner, P., & Tanner, C. (1987). Clinical judgment: How expert nurses use intuition. *American Journal of Nursing, 87*(1), 23–31.

Benner, P., & Wrubel, J. (1989). *The primacy of caring: Stress and coping in health and illness.* Menlo Park, CA: Addison-Wesley.

Carnevali, D. L., Mitchell, P. H., Woods, N. F., & Tanner, C. A. (1984). *Diagnostic reasoning in nursing.* Philadelphia: J. B. Lippincott.

Cassidy, V. R. (1987). Response changing and student achievement on objective tests. *Journal of Nursing Education, 26*(2), 60–62.

Cassidy, V. R. (1987). Test construction techniques. *Journal of Nursing Staff Development, 3*(4), 154–158.

Chenevey, B. (1988). Constructing multiple-choice examinations: Item writing. *Journal of Continuing Education in Nursing, 19*(5), 201–204.

Dell, M. S., & Valine, W. J. (1990). Explaining differences in NCLEX-RN scores with certain cognitive and noncognitive factors for new baccalaureate nurse graduates. *Journal of Nursing Education, 29*(4), 158–162.

Ebel, R. L., & Frisbie, D. A. (1986). *Essentials of educational measurement* (4th ed.). Englewood Cliffs, NJ: Prentice-Hall.

Eisenhauer, L. A., & Gendrop, S. (1990). Review of research on creative problem solving in nursing. In G. M. Clayton & P. A. Baj (Eds.), *Review of research in nursing education* (pp. 79–108). New York: National League for Nursing.

Felts, J. (1986). Performance predictors for nursing courses and NCLEX-RN. *Journal of Nursing Education, 25*(9), 372–377.

Gronlund, N. E., & Linn, R. L. (1990). *Measurement and evaluation in teaching* (6th ed.). New York: Macmillan.

Hopkins, C. D., & Antes, R. L. (1985). Classroom measurement and evaluation (2nd ed.). Itasca, IL: F. E. Peacock.

Hopkins, K. D., Stanley, J. C., & Hopkins, B. R. (1990). *Educational and psychological measurement and evaluation* (7th ed.). Englewood Cliffs, NJ: Prentice-Hall.

Litwack, L., Linc, L., & Bower, D. (1985). *Evaluation in nursing: Principles and practice.* New York: National League for Nursing.

Meyers, C. (1986). *Teaching students to think critically.* San Francisco: Jossey-Bass.

National Council of State Boards of Nursing. (1988). CAT project. *Issues, 9*(2), 4–5, 7.

National Council of State Boards of Nursing. (1989). *A research proposal for field testing CAT for nursing licensure examinations.* Chicago: Author.

Plunkett, E. J., & Olivieri, R. J. (1989). A strategy for introducing diagnostic reasoning: Hypothesis testing using a simulation approach. *Nurse Educator, 14*(6), 27–31.

Tanner, C. A. (1983). Research on clinical judgment. In W. L. Holzemer (Ed.), *Review of research in nursing education* (pp. 2–32). Thorofare, NJ: Slack.

Tanner, C. A. (1986). The nursing care plan as a teaching method: Reason or ritual? *Nurse Educator, 11*(4), 8–9.

Tanner, C. A. (1987). Teaching clinical judgment. In J. J. Fitzpatrick & R. L. Taunton (Eds.), *Annual review of nursing research* (Vol. 5, pp. 153–173). New York: Springer.

Tanner, C. A., Padrick, K. P., Westfall, U. E., & Putzier, D. J. (1987). Diagnostic reasoning strategies of nurses and nursing students. *Nursing Research, 36*(6), 358–363.

Van Ort, S., & Hazzard, M. E. (1985). A guide for evaluation of test items. *Nurse Educator, 10*(5), 13–15.

11

Methods of Evaluating Attainment of Clinical Behavioral Objectives

Teachers in a professional program such as nursing must concern themselves not only with evaluating the student's mastery of behavioral objectives as demonstrated by the usual academic procedures but also must assess the student's competency in actual practice. Professionals practice their discipline and are held accountable for the quality of their practice. Thus the development of practice competency is a critical dimension of any professional program and must be a matter of continuous evaluation.

MEANING OF CLINICAL PRACTICE

Although the term *clinical practice* is familiar to individuals involved in nursing, perceptions of the term vary considerably. To some, it implies a series or an aggregate of tasks; to others, the term implies a process.

Clinical practice may be viewed as the way or the medium through which a professional practitioner cares for clients. Clinical practice in nursing is concerned with a wide range of health problems, both actual and potential; its practitioners require a specialized body of knowledge and skills and a value system that recognizes the client as an autonomous human being with own rights. In clinical practice, the nurse uses these knowledges, skills, and values to meet the health needs of clients and contributes to the health needs of society as a whole. Practice entails competency in decision making and clinical judgment based on knowledge and intuition; caring skills, such as in the use of touch; listening and communication; treatment modalities; and moral and ethical judgment. It is through learning experiences with real situations within the practice setting that the student develops these competencies essential for professional practice.

Who are the clients? For nursing purposes, clients are individuals, groups, families, or communities. They are any of these representing all ages; any ethnic, religious, or socioeconomic group; as well as degrees of health and various stages of illness. Clients are in a variety of settings: home, community, health care facilities, schools, businesses, or industry. The nurse meets the client whenever and wherever a health need (health maintenance or illness) exists.

The nature of the relationship of nurse to client and to the problem at hand is an important consideration in defining the term *clinical practice*. Three possible views of this relationship are:

1. The nurse is in a subsidiary role, programmed as a functional agent to do things for the patient and the patient's environment. The nurse in this task-centered relationship uses prescriptions for intervention, designed for particular needs.

2. The nurse relates methods of care to the needs and problems of the client in a particular state of health. The nurse, using a nursing-process approach, views the totality of the client's being and relates professional intervention to the particular needs or problems evident in the client situation.

3. The nurse is a diagnostician, an integral part of the health service situation in which he or she intervenes. The nurse (also process-oriented) is a problem solver who develops a nursing diagnosis, proposes nursing interventions relative to the diagnosis, and carries them out through evaluation. In this relationship the nurse is involved in patient-management decisions.

Nurse teachers must develop a concept of clinical practice in terms of the nature of actions involved, the client served, and the relationship of the nurse to the clients and their problems. The concept the teacher holds determines the expectations, the evaluation strategies, and the reward systems associated with clinical practice.

PURPOSES OF CLINICAL PRACTICE IN A NURSING PROGRAM

Since nursing is a practice discipline, it requires not only cognitive mastery of relevant theories, but skill in their use within the practice domain. Practice then becomes an essential component of the preparation of the nursing practitioner and must be central to professional education, not peripheral to it.

Many of the implications of the practice component of a professional curriculum have not been carefully analyzed by nursing educators. Argyris and Schön (1974) suggest that the field experience in a professional program should not be designed simply to give students experience in the real world to learn accepted practices, but it should also provide opportunity to try out new modalities of care. Indeed, the real world may reinforce the concept of routinized practice and narrow the student's perspective of the options available to broaden and deepen one's practice.

The use of clinical practice as a means of enabling students to try out new modalities of care requires the acceptance of risk-taking behavior. This behavior is not chance behavior, but a carefully considered plan of action in which possible consequences have been identified, but the actual outcome is uncertain. It is problem-solving behavior. But can faculty support this risk-taking behavior from the students, or do they need the security of known outcome? If faculty do not accept the process of learning as well as the outcome, then they favor imitative practice and do little to encourage the creative potentials of students.

Argyris and Schön (1974) caution professional educators about the realistic misfit between the field experience and the structure of institutions of higher learning. Although they acknowledge that practice must play a central role in the process by which students learn to think like practitioners, they remind us that the school cannot claim responsibility for the preparation of all professional competencies. They state,

> The variety, duration, and realism of work experience required to provide opportunity for developing the full range of professional competencies are simply incompatible with the boundaries and structure of school experience as it is currently defined. The structure of the school year, the demands on student time made by course work, the boundaries among discipline-oriented departments, the demand of term papers and theses, the ladders of academic security and prestige all limit the intensity and duration of involvement in practice that would enable the student to acquire a full range of professional competence (p. 186).

Are the authors suggesting that faculty be more realistic in their expectations of practice competencies which the graduates are expected to achieve as they leave schools of nursing? Faculty need to explore further this misfit between the demands for acquiring clinical competence and the structural framework within which they seek to assist the learner in developing these competencies.

INFLUENCE OF THE SUPERVISORY PROCESS ON THE EVALUATION OF CLINICAL PRACTICE

Before proceeding to the discussion of strategies appropriate for clinical practice evaluation, it is important to explore the impact of the supervisory process in the clinical field on the evaluation process. The supervisory process, inherent in teaching in the practice field, generates many anxieties that differentiate evaluation of clinical practice from that of the usual academic situation.

Competency in clinical practice demands changes in behavior in all three domains (cognitive, affective, and psychomotor). Moreover, these changes must be demonstrated within the confines of a close relationship with the teacher. The process of change, which often details a period of discomfort as the new approach is being developed, occurs under the watchful eye of an observer, the teacher. Feelings of inadequacy often result, and the learner is vulnerable to fears of criticism, shame, and rejection. The degree to which these fears become operant in the student relates to the student's perception of authority. Indeed, the supervisory relationship may take on the semblance of a parent–child relationship and evoke behavioral responses commensurate with the participants' own experiences. Not only must the learner's process of becoming a practitioner occur within view of the teacher, but it usually occurs within view of many others, such as patients, families, peers, and other professionals.

In clinical evaluation, therefore, the student is even more vulnerable than in the usual educational evaluation situations. Acceptance of the realities of this vulnerability is crucial if evaluation is to be a facilitative process in the student's growth as a practitioner. A supportive climate based on trust and acceptance does much to minimize the negative effects that may result from the anxieties inherent in the evaluation of clinical practice.

If the environment is not supportive, participants in the evaluation process resort to game playing. Kadushin (1968), in his article "Games People Play in Supervision," describes many of the games that engage the energies of participants. Game playing is adopted because of the payoff. Kadushin has stated, "One party to the game chooses a strategy to maximize his payoff and minimize his penalties. He wants to win rather than to lose, and he wants to win as much as he can at the lowest cost" (p. 23).

If the learners feel threatened, they will resort to gamesmanship in an attempt to win the evaluation game. The focus of evaluation becomes survival rather than attainment of behavioral objectives relevant to clinical practice. In other words, evaluation assesses survival, not learning.

BEHAVIORS EVALUATED IN CLINICAL PRACTICE

Since the nursing process is the methodology of practice, the major focal point in evaluating the care component of clinical practice is the learner's competency in using the process. Identification of nursing actions implicit in the process, as discussed in the preceding chapter, serves as the evaluative focus. Inclusion of these behaviors does not suggest that only those behaviors directly associated with the nursing process are to be evaluated in clinical practice. Clinical practice provides opportunities for learning behaviors that pertain to the many dimensions of the professional role which are relevant to the care component but extend into other avenues where nurses function. These include:

1. *Ability to handle ambiguities as problem solving addresses real client problems and real issues of health care.*

2. *Learning how to learn as the student encounters the continuing evolution of new knowledge in the field.*

3. *Learning how professionals think at both the concrete and abstract levels.*

4. *Developing a concept of professional causation required to meet the professional and societal demands for accountability* (Reilly & Oermann, 1985, p. 406).

These behaviors are developed progressively throughout the nursing program, and their evaluation is the concern of all instructors with whom students study. Formative evaluation should reflect these behaviors as students experience more complex practice.

Nursing process behaviors are critical if the learner is to become competent in assessing the client, deriving nursing diagnoses, setting goals and planning care, intervening, and evaluating various dimensions of care. Other objectives inherent in these processes also are important. Evaluation of the student's skill in diagnostic reasoning (i.e., how the student collects data and searches for cues, generates tentative hypotheses to organize the data, decides on additional data to collect to support or reject the hypotheses, and chooses among the different alternatives available) is an important area of clinical evaluation. Objectives associated with use of knowledge and a theoretical framework in client care, interacting with clients and others in the setting, accountability, leadership and management, advocacy for nursing within the organizational structure, and other areas addressed by the program objectives represent other outcomes to be evaluated in the clinical setting. The behaviors ultimately selected for evaluation in clinical practice arise from the behavioral objectives identified for the program for which clinical practice is associated.

METHODS OF EVALUATING CLINICAL PRACTICE

When the expression *clinical practice* is used in nursing, there is a direct association with an Evaluation Form. The question usually raised is: What one form is best for clinical evaluation? It is interesting that one does not hear the question: What one form is appropriate for class evaluation?

Clinical practice is complex and cannot be evaluated by any single procedure. No form by itself is an appropriate evaluative device. The nature of the practice to be assessed is determined by the level of practice expected by the particular type of practitioner involved. If professional practice is the goal, evaluative procedures must discriminate between theoretically based practice and that which is imitative. Since the cognitive, affective, and psychomotor domains are encompassed in practice, strategies must be used to insure mastery in all domains.

As with any evaluation, the procedure used is that which provides data relative to the student's progress toward, or attainment of, specified behavioral objectives. Both summative and formative evaluation strategies are in order. However, since clinical practice competency is a developmental process, it is particularly important that a systematic approach to formative evaluation be incorporated into the program.

The focus of clinical practice evaluation is the *student*—and that student's growth toward mastery of practice; thus any evaluation procedure that provides data for making judgments about the student's practice is appropriate. Many evaluation strategies discussed in earlier chapters are suitable, especially those related to problem solving, with or without the added dimensions supplied by various forms of multimedia. Pencil-and-paper tests and written assignments also are useful in determining the cognitive base of student practice and the beliefs and values guiding student responses to the demands of practice. Evaluation procedures particularly appropriate for clinical practice may be categorized in the following three major classifications:

1. Observation.
2. Written communication.
3. Oral communication.

OBSERVATION METHODS

One of the evaluative procedures of the practice dimension of student learning used most often is observation of student behavior during nursing actions. Through observation, judgments may be made regarding cognitive, psychomotor, and affective performance. There are two components to any observation in the clinical field: (a) the specific behaviors observed (i.e., data) and (b) the inference or judgment (i.e., interpretation of these behaviors). The observation of the student's performance provides the data for evaluation; judgments may then be made based on these observations in terms of the criteria established by teacher, student, or both. It is important in clinical evaluation that sufficient data be collected before a judgment or inference is made regarding performance; different interpretations often may be made of the same data.

Observing student performance in the clinical field, as a basis for evaluation, creates the need for the teacher to be aware of own values and biases which may influence the observation and judgments made of performance. Faculty may "see different things" in any observation, as may students. Observations should be directed toward specific objectives which are known to both teacher and student. Another problem associated with observation as an evaluation method pertains to the need for observing behavior over a period of time. Because any observation is merely a sampling of behavior, the data collected may or may not be representative of true performance. As a result, behavior should be observed over a period of time or data obtained through multiple evaluation strategies before drawing conclusions about the student's performance in the clinical field.

Methods of documenting the behaviors observed in clinical practice are:

1. Anecdotal note.
2. Critical incident.
3. Rating scale.
4. Videotape.

Anecdotal Note

Anecdotal notes are frequently used in nursing education for recording data about the student's practice, although many nurse teachers have reservations about their validity and reliability. The concerns expressed relate to the format of the note, the system of collecting the notes, and the use made of the information collected.

Perhaps some teachers expect too much from anecdotal notes simply because they do not fully understand their function. An anecdotal note is a recorded description of the behavior and activities of the learner during a particular performance of short duration. It is a vignette of the learner's practice experience. The note itself is usually written informally without modifying expressions and contains only data that clarify the image of the event.

Some individuals enlarge the scope of the anecdotal note by including an interpretation or by making inferences from the event. If interpretation is desired, it should be included in a notation separate from the description and provision should be made for the learner to include a personal interpretation.

The system to be used in collecting anecdotal notes causes much concern among nurse teachers, primarily because most attempts result in an erratic pattern. Generally speaking, faculty may end up with many notes for some students (especially students having difficulty) and few notes for others, with inequities among students in the behaviors selected for recording and inconsistencies in the numbers of notes collected during various periods in the practice term. Indeed, the quantity and quality of notes may reflect the values, biases, mood and interest of the evaluator. They also neglect the influence of factors such as time and other demands being made upon the evaluator.

Many of these problems can be eliminated if a systematic approach is developed for the collection of anecdotal notes. When behavioral objectives are identified for clinical practice, nurse teachers should make decisions as to how each is to be evaluated. At that time, certain behaviors can be selected for evaluation by anecdotal notes, and the number of notes to be selected for each student can be stated. Thus, all students will be evaluated on the same behavioral objectives by the same number of notes. This system also helps the faculty to be realistic about the number of notes it is possible to collect in any clinical practice period. This decision by no means limits the number of notes a teacher may write. The teacher can still use own professional judgment about the need to obtain more data about some students. The student, however, should be informed about the increase in the number of anecdotal notes to be written and should know the rationale underlying the decision.

ILLUSTRATIONS

BEHAVIORAL OBJECTIVE	EVALUATION
A3.2 Assumes responsibility for explaining procedures to a school age child before beginning the task.	In observations recorded in anecdotal notes; the student explains the procedure.

Criteria for evaluation
1. Explanation precedes the start of the procedure
2. Explanation is in language understandable to the child
3. Explanation is accurate
4. Child is encouraged to ask questions and express concerns
5. Questions are answered accurately and sensitively

P4.0 Uses auscultation technique accurately.	In observations recorded in anecdotal notes, the student uses auscultation technique accurately.

Criteria for evaluation
1. Identifies the proper landmark
2. Uses stethoscope properly
3. Distinguishes sounds correctly
4. Carries out procedure within a reasonable time frame

These two illustrations demonstrate a use for anecdotal notes. The anecdotes are recorded, and the teacher and learner evaluate recorded behaviors according to stated criteria. This process is most effective for formative evaluation, but anecdotal notes may also be used in summative evaluation.

Anecdotal notes are valuable in recording longitudinal data about the student's progress in developing practice competency. However, there must be a systematic plan so that there are no gaps in recording, for a sufficient number of notes must be collected at regular intervals to describe the developmental process accurately. The quantitative demands of this approach, especially if large numbers of students are involved, often impede the data gathering necessary for making qualitative judgments of a student's performance ability.

Critical Incident Technique

This technique was discussed in the previous chapter as a method of assessing the student's analytic and problem-solving competencies. In the practice area, the critical incident involving some aspect of the student's performance can be recorded and performance evaluated according to stated criteria.

The concept of a critical incident differs from that of an anecdote. In a critical incident, behaviors are analyzed in terms of their effect on outcomes of the activity (Reilly & Oermann, 1985, p. 308). Anecdotes, on the other hand, are not selected because they have implications for outcome, but because they are relevant to the behavior being evaluated.

Use of the critical incident technique as a data gathering mechanism could be similar to that for the anecdotal record. Specific behavioral objectives would be identified as particularly amenable to evaluation by critical incident. The criteria for analysis of incidents, however, would be stated also in terms of student behaviors influencing outcomes of the activity positively or negatively.

ILLUSTRATION

BEHAVIORAL OBJECTIVE	EVALUATION
C3.0 Shares own assessment of patient needs with nursing colleagues	Two critical incident reports from patient care conferences. *Criteria for evaluation* 1. Identify 　a. learner behaviors which assisted nurses in understanding patient needs 　b. learner behaviors which interfered with nurses' understanding of patient needs

The critical incident technique is effective for formative evaluation; it enables the learner and the teacher to assess the learner's behaviors in relation to their impact on the outcome of an action. It can also be used in summative evaluation, provided several critical incidents are used to judge the student's mastery of the behavior under consideration.

Rating Scale

Rating scales continue to be a part of the evaluation process for nursing practice in many situations. Unfortunately, rating scales have been misused and have often been *the* method used to evaluate practice, to the exclusion of other strategies. When the request for a form for practice evaluation is made, it is often a search for a rating scale. The impossible search continues for the one perfect rating scale, which infallibly will convey the degree of competency the practitioner has achieved.

It is important to know what is meant by a rating scale. Technically, it is a standardized device for recording qualitative and quantitative judgments about *observed* performance. It may contain a list of traits, activities, skills, or attitudes that may or may not be stated behaviorally. The evaluator is asked to rate, according to best judgment, the learner's competency for each item on some point on a continuum, such as excellent-poor, achieved-not achieved and above average to below average. In general, rating scales with behaviorally expressed items are more helpful than those with items expressed as a list of traits; the behaviors are less ambiguous and relate more clearly to the course and program objectives.

Rating scales have certain limitations that must be considered when a practice evaluator is determining their use within a program. Since the scales are standardized procedures, the items (behaviors) listed may or may not be consistent with stated objectives for a particular course or learning experience. The teacher must analyze the behaviors in relation to their relevancy to objectives being evaluated, so that the rating scale selected will include statements of behaviors that at least approximate expected outcomes of the learning experience. Some behaviors on the scale may be discounted if they are not relevant.

Another limitation is the lack of uniformity with which terms are interpreted by evaluators. This is particularly true with terms used to designate various intervals in the rating continuum. An operational definition that includes illustrations of acceptable behaviors for each interval can facilitate reliability.

One of the major limitations reflects the interests and values of evaluators. Since some form of "checking off" is called for, some evaluators tend to place checks in some intervals without really doing the essential appraisal. The checking may represent a halo effect whereby the evaluator selects an interval on the continuum on the basis of prior knowledge, personal biases, or close identification with the learner. Scales that call for supportive statements to justify the interval selection help to decrease this halo effect.

The items themselves may limit the use of rating scales since they usually represent the multidimensional character of practice and all items may not be of equal importance. Thus, the value inconsistency among the items in the scale make it difficult to use the scale quantitatively.

Rating scales do have an important place in the schema for practice evaluation. They represent descriptive data of performance that suggest areas of strengths and weaknesses. They may be employed to rate an observed performance or they may be used as a summary description of performance. If used to rate an observed performance, it is important that each learner be rated more than once, for the pattern, rather than one single episode, of behavior is significant. Used in this manner, a record is made of what the learner does; the scale does not discriminate among theoretically based, imitative, and intuitive behaviors.

Rating scales, however, can be most effective in presenting data about all aspects of student practice at periodic intervals. Faculty could even devise their own rating scale from behaviors they have specified for a program, course, or unit of study. Used in this fashion, the rating scale provides a profile of student performance during regularly scheduled time periods. Such a profile is a useful tool in helping the learner as well as the teacher identify areas of practice to be supported or to be strengthened as it portrays a student's developmental progress.

Rating scales are evaluative devices that are addressed to a composite of rather than to one specific behavior. They are most effective in the system for formative evaluation. Due to irregularities in the value of different items, rating scales ordinarily are not properly subject to the grading process.

Videotape

Another strategy for recording an observation of student performance is through videotaping. Many types of behaviors may be videotaped in a variety of settings. Videotaping is advantageous because it can be played back immediately after the activity and also at a later time. Both teacher and student can then critique the performance as well as observe its development over time. Videotaping can create a vicarious experience for learners; a videotape can present a simulated situation in which students participate and then analyze. A videotape may be used to present a clinical problem, some aspect of an interpersonal encounter, or a simulated situation for critique by students (de Tornyay & Thompson, 1987) and to record the student's performance in response to the situation presented.

With videotaping students may be asked to role play and perform as they would in the clinical field. Evaluation of the performance by the student, peers, and teacher can result in significant feedback to improve not only the student's future performance but contribute to the learning of the entire group of students. Matthews and Viens (1988) describe a strategy for using videotaping for evaluating students' ability to assess and carry out an intervention. They present to the students data about a client. Students then select the role of nurse, patient, or evaluator and are videotaped on their performance. Plunkett and Olivieri (1989) propose using simulations to teach diagnostic reasoning. Client data are presented in a vignette; students work in pairs with one student assuming the role of client and the other of nurse. The vignette and subsequent role play may be videotaped which would clearly depict the client situation and provide a recording of the student's performance for immediate feedback.

Along with presenting a clinical situation in which students act out care, videotapes may be used to record a specific learner behavior or action, in the learning laboratory or clinical field, allowing for evaluation of that performance. Videotaping is an effective way of evaluating a student's ability to conduct an interview and communicate effectively with others. Students can interview a peer followed by evaluation of that interview by student, teacher and other students. Videotaping provides immediate feedback on performance and allows students to see and hear their communication with others. For psychomotor objectives, performance of skills may be videotaped for evaluation by both students and teacher to identify areas of strength and weakness and determine where more practice is needed. Students can review the videotape to more clearly critique their own performance and monitor their development of skill.

When videotaping is done in the clinical field, for instance, if the student is teaching a group of patients, protocols of the agency related to patients' privacy and other rights must be adhered to. Videotapes are particularly effective for formative evaluation but also may be used in summative evaluation for grading of performance.

WRITTEN COMMUNICATION METHODS

Nurses communicate among themselves and with practitioners of other disciplines in writing. Various forms of written communication serve as significant evaluation strategies. In this type of evaluation, one is concerned with two dimensions: skill in communicating and quality of the content communicated. Strategies for clinical evaluation include:

1. Nursing notes.
2. Nursing care plan.

3. Case study.
4. Process recording.
5. Other written assignments. Selected illustrations are included.

Nursing Notes

The ability to report and record nursing actions is identified as a critical behavior in most nursing programs. The medium for most of this reporting and recording, the patient's chart, may be used in evaluating learner competency in this area. Nursing notes may be judged in terms of their content and the student's skill in recording. Nursing notes enable faculty to evaluate the learner's ability to collect and record appropriate data about the client, state nursing diagnoses, develop and revise as indicated plans of care, and document client progress. Criteria for evaluating nursing notes include accuracy, relevance, and comprehensiveness of the data collected; accuracy in interpretation of the data; relevance of the plans of care to data analysis and goals; relevance of the interventions to the goals of care; and accuracy of the evaluation. Skill in communication reflects the student's ability to record data clearly, concisely, with proper terminology, and in a logical order.

The introduction of computers has and will continue to alter the process for documenting nursing care. Nursing information systems (NIS) use computer technology to support the delivery of patient care, including the recording of patient information and accessing relevant patient data via a computer terminal placed strategically in the nurses' station or at the patient's bedside (Brown, 1991). With use of a NIS, documentation of nursing care is accomplished on the computer rather than handwritten in a chart. Progress notes can be edited while they are being entered, although they cannot be changed after that point. Specific information about a patient, such as vital signs, intake and output, and other data often recorded on a flow sheet, can be entered into the computerized patient record. McKinney (1989) reports that nurses are more organized and efficient when computer terminals are located at each bedside, particularly in terms of charting medications and obtaining lab results. Many computer systems provide a directory of standardized care plans that can be generated from the system and then modified to reflect individual client needs.

In the community setting, care in the home can also be supported by nursing information systems. These systems can maintain client records, manage financial activities of community health and home health agencies, and improve documentation of care (Saba, 1988). In addition, nursing care planning programs as indicated above may be used to facilitate the development of care plans.

Nursing care, which is process oriented, requires considerable intradisciplinary and interdisciplinary communication so that the integrity and continuity of patient care can be maintained. Therefore, the student's communication behavior should be evaluated systematically. The evaluation of nursing notes may include several longitudinal studies in which the student's recordings of a patient are analyzed over a period of time, or it may represent a certain number of recordings of patients at a particular interval in the learning experience. The design used depends on the objective of the experience.

Nursing Care Plan

Nursing care plans are valuable for instruction and evaluation. Care plans, which enable the student to analyze the client's problems and plan related nursing management, may represent the practice model or may be prepared using a form developed by faculty. The number of care plans to be written by students depends on the learning needs of the particular student. When the evaluation data indicate the student's understanding of scientific rationale, related concepts and theories, and the fit between data and nursing action, the student should move into development of care plans which reflect the model used in the setting. This strategy enables the student to integrate more effectively nursing care plans within the total care provided to the client. Nursing care plans may be evaluated in terms of their content as well as clarity in presenting the information, use of proper terminology, conciseness of presentation, and format.

Nursing care plans relate to the assessment and planning steps of the nursing process and provide a means for evaluating the student's ability to analyze data, resulting in a nursing diagnosis, and develop a plan of care consistent with the diagnosis and individualized needs of a client. The focus of evaluation relates to the student's ability to:

Assess data in terms of relevancy to the client situation.

Interpret data consistent with a theoretical framework and considering the individuality of the client.

Cluster data and draw inferences as to their meaning.

Derive a nursing diagnosis(es) compatible with data analysis.

Prioritize nursing problems.

Select appropriate nursing interventions.

Nursing care plans as educational experiences are usually developed in a column format where horizontal relationships are evident, although some may be written in a narrative format. Column formats exhibit the relationships among the elements in the process but do not foster creative management of these elements. Plans are primarily written and submitted for evaluation. The difficulty in evaluating care plans in terms of the areas identified earlier is that the written plan itself may or may not represent the student's own critical thought processes. Instead the care plan developed by a student for a particular client may reflect the existing plan in the setting or may have been developed predominantly from the literature without sufficient consideration and analysis of the specific data base.

Whether or not care plans promote the development of critical thinking and skill in diagnostic reasoning is yet to be answered through research. Tanner (1986) indicates from a review of the research in nursing that there is no "empiric evidence to support continued reliance on the written nursing care plan as the predominant instructional method, nor is there evidence to eliminate it entirely" (p. 9). For this reason a more dynamic use of care plans occurs when these plans are presented verbally and subject to discussion and peer review. Discussion can focus on the critical thinking process underlying the resulting care plan. Students can discuss their interpretation of data, cues identified in the data, and how they were clustered; present hypotheses formulated from the data and others considered but then rejected; and describe how they arrived at decisions as to which diagnoses to support and which to reject. Similar discussion can occur as to the nursing interventions. With this strategy, the student's thinking process becomes more apparent and more readily evaluated. A combination of both approaches would be more meaningful.

Nursing care plans are an integral part of nursing management of clients. The format used in educational programs must be seen as a learning strategy and evaluated in that light. The detail required is not incorporated in the practice model in clinical settings. Therefore, it is important that the student move from the learning model to the practice model as soon as faculty are assured that the thinking competency required in managing and obtaining meaning from data is achieved. If the use of nursing care plans is prolonged beyond the learning need, they become busy work for both student and teacher.

How many nursing care plans should be developed by students in a nursing program? The key variable in responding to this question is the learning value of the experience. That factor is dependent upon the ability of each student, some requiring very few, others requiring multiple experiences. As the student progresses in the program and assumes greater responsibility for client care, the ability to plan care can be inferred from the care which the student provides. Trends portend wide use of computers for developing and communicating nursing care plans, and it is this practice skill that will become paramount.

Nursing care plans in the learning model are time-consuming for student and for faculty who carry out the evaluation, whether for formative or summative purposes. Therefore, their use and frequency of use must be justified in terms of the learning value and time allocation.

Case Study

Evaluation of a case study is particularly valuable in judging the student's ability to present a holistic concept of nursing care. The student's written description of actions implicit in meeting patient needs enables the evaluator to determine ability not only in cognitive and affective domains for each step of the process but the ability to establish meaningful relationships among steps of the process. The complexity of the problem situation in terms of nursing judgments and decisions is determined by the level of behaviors expressed for the experiences. A study designed at a comprehensive level calls for interpretative and extrapolative behaviors—behaviors very different from those required at the analytic level.

In selecting a case study method for the learner, it must be certain that the nature of the problem to be addressed and the number of variables with which the learner must deal are within the student's educational level. This means that behavioral objectives must be clearly stated and relevant to behavioral objectives of the course or unit of study. Evaluation, as with other forms of written communications, is in terms of substance and skill in the communication technique.

Modifications of the nursing case study should be encouraged so that the learner does not view the study as an end rather than as a means to an end. Other forms of problem-solving strategies, as discussed in the previous chapter, can be used to modify the case study, providing the problem is derived from the student's practice experience.

Process Recording

A procedure that has an important place in any systematic scheme for formative evaluation is the nursing process recording. The evaluative approach is directed toward the learner's behaviors in interactions with others. A process recording provides written information on the student's skill in interacting with clients and others in the clinical field.

Process recording is amenable to any interaction of the learner with another individual, such as the learner and client, the learner and a health-team member, and between learner and learner. The most frequent use for the process recording is in nurse-patient interactions.

There are various formats for recording such communications, but in general there are four main components:

1. Client communication.
2. Nurse communication.
3. Nurse's interpretation of patient communication.
4. Implications of the communication for nursing actions.

Nursing Process Recording

Client Communication	Nurse Communication	Nursing Interpretation	Implications for Nursing Actions

Client communication includes a verbatim report of all verbal and non-verbal behaviors of the client. The nurse's communication includes verbatim verbal and nonverbal behaviors of the nurse, inclusive of conscious feelings and actions. Nursing interpretation states what the nurse perceives as the client's feelings and the meanings of verbal and nonverbal actions. Implications for nursing actions are derived from the nurse's judgment of the meaning of the client's as well as his or her own communication.

A process recording is best used in conjunction with the individual conference approach, so that the teacher and the learner can evaluate the total interaction as well as each of its component parts. This procedure is especially suitable for formative evaluation, for it is carried out during the learning process and provides for diagnosis and remedial measures.

The total procedure is a time-consuming one and therefore the quantity per learning experience needs to be kept within reasonable limits. The behavioral objective(s) must be sharply defined so that the student focuses on the interaction. The report should be written immediately after the interaction occurs, while the event is vivid in the learner's memory. The teacher's evaluation and the conference should be held within a short time (at the most one week) after the event, so the learner can use the assessment in the development of interpersonal relations skills.

ILLUSTRATION

BEHAVIORAL OBJECTIVE	EVALUATION PROCEDURE
A3.3 Encourages the patient to express fears and concerns about impending surgery.	Process recording of nurse-patient interaction in the preoperative period.

Criteria for evaluation

C3.0 Identifies verbal and nonverbal clues of patient.

C3.0 Relates nursing actions to identified patient clues.

1. Identification of patient verbal and nonverbal cues
2. Identification of own verbal and nonverbal cues
3. Appropriateness of interpretation of patient behaviors
4. Relevancy of implications for nursing actions to cues exhibited in the communications

Process recording, when used with the individual conference, enables the learner to gain skill in analyzing the interaction in terms of the elements. As this skill is developed to a competency level, the learner becomes adept at recognizing inconsistencies and misunderstandings in a communication. This evaluative process is particularly effective in assisting learners to identify their own patterns of behavior in an interaction and thus to become self-evaluative about individual interpersonal relationship skills.

Other Written Assignments

Written assignments completed by students related to their practice experiences may be included in the system for clinical evaluation. Evaluation of written assignments focuses on the substantive content area of the assignment and skill in writing. Many types of written assignments may be evaluated. A teaching plan for a client, although part of the nursing process since teaching is a significant nursing intervention, may be developed separately as a learning experience to evaluate the student's ability to assess learning needs and develop a plan consistent with the needs identified; the knowledge base, health status, cultural background, and other characteristics of the client; and concepts of learning and teaching. Teaching plans also may be developed for teaching groups of clients with varied health problems and for health promotion.

Learning log and diary provide data on the learner's perceptions of the clinical experience and progress in meeting the objectives. Both of these strategies give the teacher a view of learning from the student's own perspective. Because of the nature of logs and diaries, they are most suitable for formative evaluation.

Other types of written assignments which may be evaluated as part of the clinical evaluation include: reports of observations made in the clinical agency in which students practice and in other settings, papers which analyze a specific clinical experience, analyses of clinical decisions, position papers on moral and ethical issues which arise in the clinical setting, a comparative study of two or more client responses to a similar health phenomenon, an analysis of the process of staff decision making regarding a plan of care for a client, and an examination of the cultural values of a client and family and impact on care.

ORAL COMMUNICATION METHODS

Nurses communicate not only through the written media, but they must also be able to convey their ideas and thinking through the spoken word. This ability is of particular importance when presenting information or sharing in the decision-making process with intraprofessional and interprofessional colleagues. Evaluation methods that provide data on the learner's ability to communicate verbally are

1. Clinical conferences.
2. Nursing and multidisciplinary conferences.

Clinical Conferences

Clinical conferences take various forms, but in general they are problem-solving group discussions about some facet of clinical practice. In one format, the student represents a patient situation to the peer group for critical analysis of the plan of action or its implication. The peers evaluate the actions, raise relevant questions, and propose appropriate alternatives. In some instances the conferences may be preceded by nursing rounds in which participants have the opportunity to observe the patients whose nursing care will be discussed.

Other conferences may be less structured and obtain substance from the learner's activities of the day. In this conference format, problems with which the learners are currently engaged are presented for group participation in proposing solutions.

Regardless of format, when group conferences are used in the evaluation schema, the teacher is concerned not only with the quality of the substance and the skillful use of communication techniques (as with written communication methods), but also with the learner's ability to use the group process. Nursing for the most part involves groups, and it is essential that behaviors relevant to individual participation in group process be identified and evaluated. The conference provides an excellent medium for formative evaluation of the student in his or her development in the skills in group work.

Conferences are primarily problem-solving experiences, and the conferences can accordingly be addressed to a particular behavioral objective or to several objectives.

ILLUSTRATIONS

BEHAVIORAL OBJECTIVES

C4.2   Relates the plan of nursing action to the hospitalized patient's adaptive response to stress.

C3.0   Uses leadership principles in assisting the conference members to reach nursing managerial decisions.

EVALUATION PROCEDURE

Nursing Care Conference
1. Student presentation of the stress-adaptation phenomenon as operant in a hospitalized patient
2. Student leadership of group in arriving at nursing managerial decisions

Criteria for evaluation
1. Clarity and comprehensiveness of the identification of stressors
2. Accuracy and completeness of the explanation of demands placed on the patient by these stressors
3. Clarity and comprehensiveness of the identification of patient adaptive behavior
4. Leadership in involving group members in managerial decisions
5. Relevance of decisions to the patient's adaptive response

The clinical conference is a valuable evaluation strategy and may be used as either a formative or a summative evaluation procedure.

Nursing and Multidisciplinary Conferences

These conferences are other types of small group activities that serve as an effective strategy in evaluating clinical practice. The composition of participants may vary, ranging from a nursing group of practitioners in a particular clinical setting to a highly organized multidisciplinary team in a health care agency or in a community. The definition of membership is also variable. In some situations, a health team is composed of health care professionals only; in other situations patients and/or community representatives are included as health-team members.

Whatever the composition of the team, the process in which it is engaged is essentially the same: shared managerial decision making. The learner's participation may range from a sharing process to the highly developed skill of collaboration. The nature of the participation is determined by the stated behavioral objective for the experience.

The most common group activity is problem solving in which, through group process, plans for patient care are developed according to stated patient goals. Implementation of the plan is examined and evaluated for its effectiveness. The learner is evaluated in terms of participation in the group in reporting observations, drawing relationships among data, making proposals for action, and evaluating actions as they are reported.

ILLUSTRATION

BEHAVIORAL OBJECTIVE

C4.3   Collaborates with nursing colleagues in managerial decisions for a patient.

EVALUATION PROCEDURE

Nursing Conference
Presentation to nurses in a clinical setting, a patient situation necessitating decisions for a plan for management.

Criteria for evaluation
1. Collects data from other nurses
2. Reports own observations
3. Shares with group in interpreting data
4. Shares with group in establishing relationships among data
5. Provides for all members to contribute ideas relative to goals for care
6. Leads group to consensus of goals

BEHAVIORAL OBJECTIVE   EVALUATION PROCEDURE

                                         7. Listens to members' suggestions for implementation strategies

                                         8. Develops plan of care for patient relevant to needs on the basis of group consensus

Evaluative data about the student in the situation described above may be obtained through the evaluator's observation of the student's behavior, through evaluation reports submitted by the students and other participants, through study of a tape recording, or through a videotape of the conference. The results of the evaluation may be used in formative or summative evaluation.

MULTIPLE APPROACHES TO CLINICAL EVALUATION

This chapter has dealt with some of the possible strategies that may be used in evaluating the learner's practice. Actually the extent of the range of strategies is limited only by the teacher's creativity and willingness to take risks and become innovative.

One of the greatest dangers in clinical evaluation is the tendency of the teacher to "get into a rut" with evaluation procedures and to use the same process in each evaluation period with every student. As the approach becomes routinized, practice evaluation becomes an end in itself, divorced from the excitement of learning.

Behavioral objectives, as described and used in this book, are open-ended to encourage teachers to develop their own evaluation strategies. The following example illustrates several approaches that may be used to evaluate a particular behavioral objective.

ILLUSTRATION

BEHAVIORAL OBJECTIVE   EVALUATION METHODS

C3.0 Conducts purposeful   *Possible Approaches*
interviews.   1. Observation by the evaluator
                                         2. Tape recording
                                         3. Videotaping
                                         4. Written interview report
                                         5. Clinical conference

BEHAVIORAL OBJECTIVE   EVALUATION METHODS

Criteria for evaluation
1. Clear definition of purpose
2. Questions related to purpose
3. Questions stated to elicit
   responses relevant to purpose
4. Questions comprehensive in scope
5. Responses of patient consistent
   with scope
6. Patient cues acknowledged
7. Nurse's evaluation of interview in
   terms of principles of interviewing

It will be noted that five evaluation strategies for the single behavioral objective are suggested. The teacher can vary the strategies with different groups of students, so that they are not confined to one method and thus run the risk of becoming bored and automatic in the preparation of evaluation reports. The suggestion of the five methods is especially important, however, in enabling the teacher to individualize evaluation procedures. Different methods may be used with different students, according to their needs and the situation in which they are practicing.

Although educators profess a belief in individualized learning, they generally require all students to "march to the same drummer" as far as evaluation is concerned. A teacher who adopts a mastery-of-learning approach does not conclude that a student is incapable of meeting the objective on the basis of performance on one evaluation strategy. In the illustration, if the written report of the interview is selected as the evaluation strategy and a student's report is unacceptable, should one then conclude that the student is incapable of conducting a purposeful interview? A mastery-of-learning teacher would select another evaluation procedure before drawing such a conclusion. Perhaps a tape recording or a videotape of an interview would provide evidence that the student could meet the objective.

The suggestion here is that teachers recognize the complex nature of practice and accordingly diversify their evaluation strategies so that the learner and the teacher engage in a developmental rather than a controlling process.

SUMMARY

Evaluation of the learner's clinical practice is a critical element in professional educational programs. The practice of professionals is a complex process by which they care for clients. Nursing process is the methodology of nursing practice and represents a composite of cognitive, affective, and psychomotor behaviors. Clinical practice within a nursing education program serves many purposes which must be recognized by faculty.

Evaluation of the learner's practice skills occurs in an environment with built-in threats and pressures. Not only does the supervisory process, by its nature, generate anxieties, but the process takes place in an environment that makes the learner particularly vulnerable. The developmental process that changes behavior takes place in full view of patients, colleagues, and other health workers. Care must be taken that game playing is not resorted to as a means of lessening threats in the clinical field.

The multiplicity of abilities called upon in effective nursing practice demands diverse clinical evaluation strategies. No one procedure is suitable for assessing the totality of practice. Strategies chosen should reflect the particular behavioral objectives to be evaluated, the needs of the learner, and the character of the practice setting.

Procedures appropriate for clinical practice evaluation include:

1. Observation (anecdotal note, critical incident, rating scale, and videotape).

2. Written communication (nursing notes, nursing care plan, case study, process recording, and other written assignments).

3. Oral communication (clinical, nursing, and multidisciplinary conferences).

REFERENCES

Argyris, C., & Schön, D. (1974). A theory in practice: Increasing professional effectiveness. San Francisco: Jossey-Bass.

Brown, P. A. (1991). Computers in nursing practice. In M. H. Oermann, Professional nursing practice: A conceptual approach. Philadelphia: J. B. Lippincott.

de Tornyay, R., & Thompson, M. A. (1987). Strategies for teaching nursing (3rd ed.). New York: John Wiley & Sons.

Kadushin, A. (1968, July). Games people play in supervision. Social Work, 13, 23–32.

Matthews, R., & Viens, S. (1988). Evaluating basic nursing skills through group video testing. Journal of Nursing Education, 27(1), 44–46.

McKinney, P. (1988). Can point of care terminals ease the threat? Computers in Healthcare, 9(4), 62.

Plunkett, E. J., & Olivieri, R. J. (1989). A strategy for introducing diagnostic reasoning: Hypothesis testing using a simulation approach. Nurse Educator, 14(6), 27–31.

Reilly, D. E., & Oermann, M. H. (1985). Clinical field: Its use in nursing education. Norwalk, CT: Appleton-Century-Crofts.

Saba, V. K. (1988). Taming the computer jungle of NISs. *Nursing & Health Care, 9*(9), 487–491.

Tanner, C. A. (1986). The nursing care plan as a teaching method: Reason or ritual? *Nurse Educator, 11*(4), 8–9.

RECOMMENDED READINGS

American Nurses' Association. (1973). *Standards of nursing practice.* Kansas City: Author.

Beare, P. (1985). The clinical contract—An approach to competency-based clinical learning and evaluation. *Journal of Nursing Education, 24*(2), 75–77.

Bizek, K. S., & Oermann, M. H. (1990). Study of educational experiences, support, and job satisfaction among critical care nurse preceptors. *Heart & Lung, 19,* 439–444.

Bondy, K. N. (1983). Criterion-referenced definitions for rating scales in clinical evaluation. *Journal of Nursing Education, 22,* 376–382.

Bondy, K. N. (1984). Clinical evaluation of student performance: The effects of criteria on accuracy and reliability. *Research in Nursing and Health, 7,* 25–33.

Bongartz, C. (1988). Computer-oriented patient care. *Computers in Nursing, 6*(5), 204–210.

Burns, K. A. (1984). Experience in the use of gaming and simulation as an evaluation tool for nurses. *Journal of Continuing Education in Nursing, 15*(5), 213–217.

Clayton, G. M., Broome, M. E., & Ellis, L. A. (1989). Relationship between a preceptorship experience and role socialization of graduate nurses. *Journal of Nursing Education, 28*(2), 72–75.

Eisenhauer, L. A., & Gendrop, S. (1990). Review of research on creative problem solving in nursing. In G. M. Clayton & P. A. Baj (Eds.), *Review of research in nursing education* (pp. 79–108). New York: National League for Nursing.

Fried, A. K., Killion, V. J., & Schick, L. C. (1988). Computerized databases in nursing. *Computers in Nursing, 6*(6), 244–252.

Goldsmith, J. W. (1984). Effect of learner variables, media attributes, and practice conditions on psychomotor task performance. *Western Journal of Nursing Research, 6*(2), 229–240.

Grabbe, L. L. (1988). A comparison of clinical evaluation tools in hospitals and baccalaureate nursing programs. *Journal of Nursing Education, 27*(9), 394–397.

Gross, M. S. (1988). The potential of information systems in nursing. *Nursing & Health Care, 9*(9), 477–479.

Higgins, B., & Ochsner, S. (1989). Two approaches to clinical evaluation. *Nurse Educator, 14*(2), 8–11.

Infante, M. S., Forbes, E. J., Houldin, A. D., & Naylor, M. D. (1989). A clinical teaching project: Examination of a clinical teaching model. *Journal of Professional Nursing, 5*(3), 132–139.

Johnson, G., Lehman, B. B., & Sandoval, N. B. (1988). Clinical exam: A summative evaluation tool. *Journal of Nursing Education, 27*(8), 373–374.

Kolb, S. E., & Shugart, E. B. (1984). Evaluation: Is simulation the answer? *Journal of Nursing Education, 23,* 84–86.

Larson, C. E. (1987). Use of the microcomputer as a tool for subjective grading. *Computers in Nursing, 5*(5), 186–191.

Leino-Kilpi, H. (1989). Learning to care—A qualitative perspective of student evaluation. *Journal of Nursing Education, 28*(2), 61–66.

Lenburg, C. B. (1979). *The clinical performance examination.* New York: Appleton-Century-Crofts.

Litwack, L., Linc, L., & Bower, D. (1985). *Evaluation in nursing: Principles and practice.* New York: National League for Nursing.

Malek, C. J. (1988). Clinical evaluation: Challenging tradition. *Nurse Educator, 13*(6), 34–37.

McKnight, J., Rideout, E., Brown, B., Ciliska, D., Patton, D., Rankin, J., & Woodward, C. (1987). The objective structured clinical examination: An alternative approach to assessing student clinical performance. *Journal of Nursing Education, 26*(1), 39–41.

Miller, M. A., & Malcolm, N. S. (1990). Critical thinking in the nursing curriculum. *Nursing & Health Care, 11*(2), 67–73.

Morgan, M. K., & Irby, D. M. (1978). *Evaluating clinical competence in the health professions.* St. Louis: Mosby.

Novak, S. (1988). An effective clinical evaluation tool. *Journal of Nursing Education, 27*(2), 83–84.

Oermann, M. H. (1984). Analyzing and selecting audio-visual materials. *Nurse Educator, 9* (4), 24–27.

Oermann, M. H. (in press). Psychomotor skill development. *Journal of Continuing Education in Nursing.*

Pagana, K. D. (1989). Psychometric evaluation of the clinical stress questionnaire. *Journal of Nursing Education, 28*(4), 169–174.

Romano, C. A. (1987). Privacy, confidentiality, and security of computerized systems: The nursing responsibility. *Computers in Nursing, 5*(3), 99–104.

Scheetz, L. J. (1989). Baccalaureate nursing student preceptorship programs and the development of clinical competence. *Journal of Nursing Education, 28*(1), 29–35.

Schwirian, P. M. (1978). Evaluating the performance of nurses: A multi-dimensional approach. *Nursing Research, 27*(6), 347–351.

Tanner, C. A. (1987). Teaching clinical judgment. In J. J. Fitzpatrick & R. L. Taunton (Eds.), *Annual review of nursing research* (Vol. 5, pp. 153–173). New York: Springer.

Tower, B. L., & Majewski, T. V. (1987). Behaviorally based clinical evaluation. *Journal of Nursing Education, 26*(3), 120–123.

van Bemmerl, J. H. (1987). Computer-assisted care in nursing. *Computers in Nursing, 5*(4), 132–139.

Wakim, J. H. (1986). Developing evaluation tools. *Nurse Educator, 11* (4), 26–30.

Waltz, C. F., & Miller, C. H. (Eds.). (1988). *Educational outcomes: Assessment of quality—A compendium of measurement tools for baccalaureate nursing programs.* New York: National League for Nursing.

Woolley, A. (1977). The long and tortured history of clinical evaluation. *Nursing Outlook, 25*(5), 308–315.

12

Behavioral Objectives and Evaluation —Accountability

The concept of instructional accountability was introduced in the beginning of this book. Inherent in this concept is the need for some type of quality control. In instructional endeavors, quality control concerns two critical dimensions: relevancy of the instruction and responsibility for the quality of the instruction. As stated in Chapter 1, instructional accountability is one aspect of program accountability. The latter also deals with such matters as the student's own evaluation, the process itself, and the determination of the rightness of objectives. Instructional accountability relates to the question of attainment or nonattainment of the stated goal of the educational experience.

NATURE OF THE RELATIONSHIP BETWEEN THE WHAT AND THE HOW

Any plan designed to ascertain the quality of the instructional effort concerns two variables: the *what* (behavioral objectives) and the *how* (evaluation strategies). These two variables, however, are not viewed as separate entities, for it is the relationship between the two variables that influences the reliability and validity of the accountability process. Precisely stated, relevant behaviors have little import if the strategies for evaluating their attainment are not appropriate. Further, well constructed and creative evaluation procedures are meaningless if not directed toward behavioral objectives designed for a particular learning endeavor.

The relationship between the *what* and the *how* is an interdependent one. When behavioral objectives for a learning experience are stated, the underlying assumption is that they will be attained by most learners. Proper testing for achievement depends on the use of appropriate evaluation processes. Evaluation strategies gain their significance from stated behavioral objectives.

Nevertheless, this relationship is not an automatic, highly structured one in which a known behavioral objective is associated with a known evaluative strategy. It cannot be diagrammed as Behavioral Objective ⟶ Evaluation Strategy, similar to the familiar Stimulus ⟶ Response diagram. Operating within this relationship are teachers and learners and all their potentials for creativity. The relationship is dynamic, responsive to novelty, change, and environmental stressors.

The relationship is also creative. The teacher and the learner are free to explore their own ideas and to interject new approaches. As long as the integrity of the relationship is maintained, the methodology for demonstrating the relationship is open to examination and to trial.

The relationship should be exciting for teacher and learner. Variety and novelty can be stimuli for involvement so that assessment of learning does not become an end in itself but an integral part of the instructional process and an opportunity for self-knowledge. When the intent of the relationship between the *what* and the *how* is clear to all participants in the instructional endeavor, the freedom to develop the relationship in a meaningful way presents a challenge. Although the teacher is ultimately held accountable for the relevance and quality of the instruction, student participation in developing the relationship between behavioral objectives and the strategies for their assessment helps the learner to recognize those aspects of the learning process for which one must be held accountable. Therefore, accountability becomes a shared responsibility, demanding specific commitment from all participants.

RELATIONSHIP OF THE CLINICAL AND THE CLASS EVALUATION OF A BEHAVIORAL OBJECTIVE

Professional education provides evaluation schema not only for the academic situation usually associated with higher education, but also for situations in which the learner can demonstrate ability in those competencies associated with the practice of a chosen profession. The two schema, however, do not imply that two separate sets of behavioral objectives are necessarily indicated. Since professional education is comprised of all three domains of learning (cognitive, affective, and psychomotor), many behavioral objectives may be evaluated in both the classroom and the practice settings.

Behavioral objectives that are open-ended provide clues to evaluation strategies but do not prescribe them. Thus the teacher and, in some cases, the learner are free to develop alternative approaches, providing they maintain the relationship of the evaluation procedure to the stated behavior.

ILLUSTRATION

BEHAVIORAL OBJECTIVE	CLASS EVALUATION	CLINICAL EVALUATION
C2.2 Describes the influence of emotions on communication.	Listen to four tapes of the interaction of two individuals. Each tape represents a dialogue characterized by one of the following emotions: love, anger, distrust, fear.	Make *two* observations of communication between a patient and a staff member or between two patients in which one of the following four emotions is present: love, anger, distrust, fear.
	Select two of the communication episodes and describe in writing the effect of the emotion on: Voice tone Content Flow of communication Ending of communication	Describe in writing the effect of emotion on: Voice tone Content Flow of communication Ending of communication

In this illustration, data relative to the student's mastery of the behavioral objective may be secured from the class setting and from the clinical setting. One evaluative approach is suggested here for each, but most readers could think of many other strategies for testing this behavior in each area. The class evaluation might be conducted in class or it might be an out-of-class assignment. The clinical evaluation is suggested as a written communication, but it could also be an oral communication in which the student could present the findings at a nursing conference. Not only could the method vary, but the task could vary. There are innumerable ways to assess this behavior and it is up to the teacher to devise different approaches. Diversity is the challenge of evaluation.

ADDITIONAL ILLUSTRATIONS

BEHAVIORAL OBJECTIVE	CLASS EVALUATION	CLINICAL EVALUATION
C4.1 Identifies feelings of an individual who has AIDS.	*Essay Question* Brian Smith, age 25, has just been told by a physician that he has AIDS. As a nurse, what feelings do you anticipate Brian will experience? Explain your rationale in terms of theories and concepts relevant to the situation.	*Nursing Conference* Presentation of a patient situation in which the nurse identifies feelings of a patient who has a diagnosis of AIDS. *Criteria* 1. Types of feelings identified 2. Supporting data 3. Completeness of assessment
C2.2 Describes the behavior of elderly people in selected situations.	*Written Assignment* Select two of the following situations and observe for 10 minutes the behavior of an elderly person in terms of: 1. Independent actions 2. Interactions with others 3. Body mannerisms Write up your observations.	Observe for 10 minutes the behavior of two elderly hospitalized patients (one, confined to bed, and the other, mobile) in terms of: 1. Independent actions 2. Interactions with others 3. Body mannerisms Report your observations at a clinical conference.

BEHAVIORAL OBJECTIVE	CLASS EVALUATION	CLINICAL EVALUATION
	Situations	
	1. On a bus	
	2. In a store	
	3. In church or synagogue	
	4. In a family group	
	5. At a social activity for the elderly	

As with the first illustrations, these two illustrations are included to show the potential for evaluating a particular behavioral objective in both settings of the students' experience—the clinical and the classroom.

PLAN FOR THE EVALUATION OF BEHAVIORAL OBJECTIVES

Teaching, learning, and evaluation all are vibrant, dynamic processes whose characteristics reflect the values, beliefs, and attitudes of participants. The first aspect of the educational process to reflect these individuals is the development of behavioral objectives for the instructional program. The behaviors indicate beliefs about the developmental process of the learner and the nature of the practice by which nurses serve the society. The content indicates the field of knowledge deemed necessary for the behaviors to be actualized.

Once the behaviors and content of the behavioral objectives are identified, planning must provide for operationalizing the behavioral objectives. At this point the character of the teaching–learning process is proclaimed, as the selection of methods and learning experiences is made on the basis of the teacher's concept of the teaching–learning process. The teacher who proposes diverse approaches to operationalizing behavioral objectives is free to individualize the learner's educational experience because options are available.

As is consistent with the concept of unified teaching and learning, the teacher devises evaluation strategies for each behavioral objective. Here, too, diversity is a key factor so that various options are available to the learner. It is to be noted that all such planning precedes the actual teaching–learning experience. Preplanning of evaluation is particularly important if the relationship between behavioral objectives and the evaluation process is to be maintained.

In too many instances teachers scurry about at evaluation time trying retrospectively to devise some type of examination. The question, "What approaches should I use to evaluate the behavioral objective?" is not the one that is asked. More often questions such as "What material was covered in class?" "Can we ask questions on the readings from the bibliography?" are heard.

When the latter questions control the teacher's development of the evaluation instrument, then the teacher does not perceive the relationship between behavioral objectives and evaluation strategies. If the relationship determines the teacher's evaluation approach, questions as to where the student developed a particular learning would be recognized as irrelevant. The primary concern is the student's mastery of the behavior stated in the objective. Because this is so, evaluation can be developed before the actual course or unit is offered. Preplanning, which also includes alternatives to meet exigencies that may arise in the situation, frees the teacher and the learner alike to devote their energies to the learning process, for both know what will be the focus of the evaluation during periods of formative and summative evaluation.

It is important to stress here that the relationship between behavioral objectives and evaluation is not absolute. Learning is a dynamic process, often resulting in unanticipated outcomes which are of significance to the development of the learner and teacher. The teacher must be alert to these new happenings and use them within the educational experience of the student.

The statement of behavioral objectives in any part of the curriculum represents the best judgment of a faculty or individual teacher as to the essential outcomes which can reasonably be achieved by most students. They provide a baseline or framework, but they are not restrictive to serendipitous experiences and learnings which arise.

The teacher is accountable to assure that learning experiences are available so as to enable students to achieve the stated intended behaviors and that evaluation will be addressed to those behaviors. Experiences which are enabling do not guarantee that achievement of competency will occur, for many factors within the student affect mastery attainment. The creative teacher is able to maximize potential learning experience that will facilitate the movement of students who so desire beyond the scope specified by the behavioral objectives.

EVALUATION AND ACCOUNTABILITY

The importance of maintaining the relationship between behavioral objectives and the evaluation process at all levels of the instructional endeavor, from the individual experience through to the overall program itself, cannot be stressed enough. If behavioral objectives are expressed within a developmental model so that each part of the system contributes to other parts and to the total system itself, then the evaluation of behavioral objectives should be developed within the context of the same model. At each point in the system, the integrity of the relationship is maintained, so that achievement of each behavioral objective can be appraised. The close and contributory interrelationship of behavioral objectives to the total system necessitates that they be evaluated at whatever level in the system they occur. Any evaluation schema that fails to provide for evaluation of each behavioral objective at every level increases risks that incomplete data will be used in making judgments about the practitioner's competency.

Consistency in maintaining the relationship between evaluation strategies and behavioral objectives is not only relevant to the evaluation of the student while in the program, but it is a vital aspect of any program for quality control. When accountability is called for, this does not mean that only the final product is subject to quality control. Each subsystem must meet the demands of accountability, for the total educational endeavor is dependent on the quality of instruction at each level in the system. A program that states behavioral objectives at each level within a developmental framework and that requires relevant evaluation strategies for each level is designed to establish accountability for its instructional endeavor.

SUMMARY

A direct relationship exists between the *what* (behavioral objectives) and the *how* (evaluation processes) of an educational endeavor. The relationship is an interdependent one whose character reflects the values and beliefs of participants.

Maintaining the integrity of the relationship is critical if the instructional endeavor is to meet the demands of quality control and if participants are to be held accountable for the quality of the outcome. The declaration of behavioral objectives, their development in a program of studies, and evaluation of their attainment are the processes of education.

Index

253